286
Current Topics
in Microbiology
and Immunology

Springer

Berlin
Heidelberg
New York
Hong Kong
London
Milan
Paris
Tokyo

I.H. Madshus (Ed.)

Signalling from Internalized Growth Factor Receptors

With 19 Figures

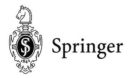 Springer

Professor Inger Helene Madshus, M.D., Ph.D.
Institute of Pathology
Rikshospitalet University Hospital
0027 Oslo
Norway

e-mail: i.h.madshus@labmed.uio.no

Cover illustration by I.H. Madshus
The receptor tyrosine kinase ErbB2 (green) is over-expressed in the breast carcinoma
cell line SKBr3. ErbB2 is endocytosis deficient and excluded from early endosome
antigen positive endosomes (blue).

ISSN 0070-217X
ISBN 3-540-21038-5
Springer-Verlag Berlin Heidelberg New York

Library of Congress Catalog Card Number 72-152360

Springer-Verlag is a part of Springer Science+Business Media
springeronline.com

© Springer-Verlag Berlin Heidelberg 2004
Printed in Germany

Editor: Dr. Rolf Lange, Heidelberg
Desk editor: Anne Clauss, Heidelberg
Production editor: Andreas Gösling, Heidelberg
Cover design: design & production GmbH, Heidelberg
Typesetting: Stürtz AG, Würzburg
Printed on acid-free paper – 27/3150 ag   5 4 3 2 1 0

Preface

Mammalian cells are to a large extent controlled by the environment. Diffusible factors (growth factors, cytokines, and hormones) released by other cells in the body bind to and activate receptors localized at the cell surface. In the case of the fibroblast growth factor receptor, there seems to be receptors both at the plasma membrane and in the nucleus. Cellular receptors control growth, apoptosis, immune function, differentiation, development, and upon dysregulation, cancer progression and metastasis. Upon ligand binding, most receptors are internalized. However, the mechanisms of endocytosis are diverse, and receptors are taken into cells from different membrane microdomains. Activation of receptors results in two important interconnected processes, namely, signal transduction and endocytosis. Interestingly, signal transduction controls endocytosis and endocytosis controls signalling. In both processes sequential formation of transient protein machineries is crucial. Currently, characterization of such complex machineries is advancing rapidly. It has recently become appreciated that several post-translational modifications directly control the affinity of protein–protein interactions. This volume of *Current Topics in Microbiology and Immunology* focuses on the recent understanding of signalling from internalized activated growth factor receptors. This includes information on pathways by which the rate and specificity of endocytosis and intracellular sorting are controlled. It further includes information on how specialized signalling and trafficking platforms are formed at the plasma membrane and on intracellular vesicles. Recent advances in cell biology and bioinformatics have revealed the existence of several conserved protein modules, such as UIM, UEV, UBA, and CUE domains, that endow proteins with the ability to bind the small, conserved peptide ubiquitin. Ubiquitination thereby turns out to be a key process in controlling affinity and specificity of protein interactions and therefore in controlling both signal transduction and intracellular transport. As discussed in the chapter by Sigismund et al., evidence is accumulating that monoubiquitination, in addition to controlling membrane trafficking of receptors, controls histone function, transcription regulation, DNA repair, and DNA replication. This opens up a new and exciting avenue in science that will eventually shed light on some of the fundamental and complex processes of cell biology.

Inger Helene Madshus

List of Contents

List of Contributors

(Their addresses can be found at the beginning of their respective chapters.)

CTMI (2004) 286:1–19

Receptor Tyrosine Kinase Signaling and Trafficking—Paradigms Revisited

M. A. Barbieri · T. P. Ramkumar · S. Fernadez-Pol · P. I. Chen ·
P. D. Stahl (✉)

Department of Cell Biology and Physiology, School of Medicine,
Washington University, 660 S. Euclid Avenue, Campus Box 8228, St. Louis,
MO 63110, USA
pstahl@cellbiology.wustl.edu

Abstract The recognition of growth factors and other cell signaling agents by their cognate cell surface receptors triggers a cascade of signal transducing events. Ligand binding and subsequent activation of many signal transducing receptors increases their rate of internalization. Endocytosis of the receptor has always been viewed as primarily a mechanism for signal attenuation and receptor degradation, but recent evidence suggests that internalization may result in the formation of specialized signaling platforms on intracellular vesicles. Thus, understanding how interactions between receptors and intracellular signaling molecules, such as adaptors, GTPases, and kinases, are regulated will undoubtedly provide insight into the ways that cells sense and adapt to the extracellular milieu.

1
Introduction

Signaling from the extracellular environment is achieved through unique, dynamic, and efficient signal transduction systems. The first cellular components that come in contact with external signals are cell surface receptors. Receptor tyrosine kinases (RTKs) constitute a large group of receptors that respond to growth factors and have intrinsic tyrosine kinase activity. On ligand binding, RTKs dimerize and, through a conformation change, intrinsic cytoplasmic kinase activity is switched on, which in turn results in autophosphorylation of the RTK (Schlessinger 2000; Neer 1995). Autophosphorylation of tyrosine residues in receptors creates binding sites for proteins containing Src-homology-2 (SH2) and phosphotyrosine-binding (PTB) domains. These interacting proteins may serve as adaptors and/or show enzymatic activities [e.g., ligand-regulated guanine nucleotide exchange factors (GEFs) that regulate the function of the particular RTK]. Alteration of either the adaptor function or the enzymatic activity may affect the cascade of protein–protein and protein–lipid interactions, phosphorylations, and dephosphorylations, and the production of secondary messengers, that lead ultimately to altered gene transcription and cellular function.

It has been observed that many RTKs are rapidly endocytosed on ligand activation, after which they traffic through the endomembrane network, an elaborate system of interconnecting tubules and vesicles that mediate the transport of fluid and selected membrane proteins. The suggestion that these endocytic membranes have a role in cell signaling has been an open question.

Cell surface receptors have also served as model systems for the study of general mechanisms and pathways of endocytic transport. Early studies of the relationship between signaling and endocytosis relied mostly on the use of subcellular fractionation of membrane compartments and on the analysis of receptors harboring mutations. More recently, experimental approaches to interfere with specific mechanisms of membrane transport have been developed, allowing a detailed study of specific signaling and membrane transport events in living cells.

In this review, we highlight the close ties between endocytosis and signaling by discussing important observations from early studies along with selected recent studies that have provocative implications.

2
Endocytosis of Signaling Receptor

The most comprehensive studies of RTK endocytosis have been carried out with the epidermal growth factor (EGF) receptor as a model system (Fig. 1). Cellular stimulation with EGF results in rapid clustering of EGF receptor complexes in clathrin-coated pits and the subsequent internalization into clathrin-coated endocytic vesicles (Gorden et al. 1978;

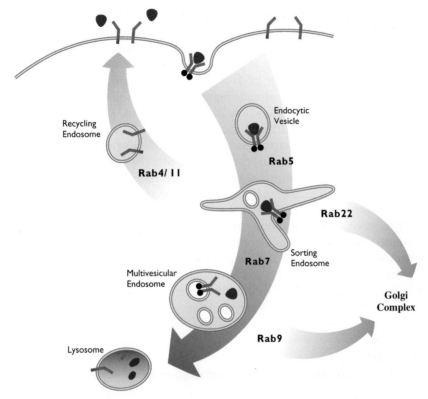

Fig. 1. Endocytic pathway: This figure shows the progression of an endocytic vesicle from internalization to maturation at the lysosome. RTKs are used to illustrate the possible fates of an endocytosed receptor complex. The various Rab GTPases thought to be involved in this pathway are also indicated. Rab22 may play a role in membrane sorting in the early endosome (Mesa et al. 2001)

Hanover et al. 1984; Carpentier et al. 1982). The internalization of EGF receptors can be effectively blocked by dominant-negative mutants of several regulatory proteins. Examples include dynamin, a cytoplasmic GTPase that is necessary for the fission of coated vesicles from the plasma membrane, and Rab5, a cytoplasmic GTPase that is necessary for endosome fusion (Barbieri et al. 2000; Damke et al. 1994; Carbone et al. 1997). Under physiological conditions, coated pits are the main routes for internalization of growth factor receptors. However, these receptors have also been shown to internalize by clathrin-independent processes that resemble micropinocytosis, particularly in cells overexpressing the receptor (Haigler et al. 1979; Hopkins et al. 1985).

Endocytosis by both clathrin-dependent and clathrin-independent mechanisms delivers receptors to early endosomes, a heterogeneous population of membrane compartments with tubular-vesicular morphology that is located mainly at the cell periphery (Hopkins et al. 1985). Receptors then either can be recycled to the plasma membrane from peripheral and perinuclear endosomes (late recycling compartment) or can progress to lysosomes, where they are degraded. Fusion of early endosomes and their centripetal movement causes internalized receptors to redistribute to compartments in the perinuclear area (Gruenberg and Maxfield 1995). These endosomes often show a characteristic morphology of multivesicular endosomes (MVEs), also referred to as multivesicular bodies—large membrane compartments that contain smaller vesicles in their lumen (McKanna et al. 1979; Miller et al. 1986). RTKs that are not recycled to the membrane after endocytosis (Sorkin et al. 1991) are retained in endosomes and accumulate in both the limiting and internal membranes of MVEs (Miller et al. 1986; Sorkin et al. 1991; Felder et al. 1990). The process of inward invagination of an MVE membrane is thought to trap receptors in the MVE interior, which prevents recycling and promotes their delivery to lysosomes.

3
Receptor Trafficking: Endocytic Regulation of Signaling Pathways

It is clear that activation of RTKs like EGF receptor and insulin receptor can stimulate receptor internalization. Receptor activation may also have secondary effects on general membrane dynamics. One of the earliest reported effects of EGF in membrane trafficking was the stimulation of membrane ruffling and macropinocytosis (Haigler et al. 1979). A rapid increase in fluid-phase endocytosis has been observed in response to EGF and insulin stimulation, but the internalization rates of cargo receptors, such as transferrin receptor, do not appear to be affected (Haigler et al. 1979; Wiley and Cunningham 1982). There is some evidence to suggest that this "increase" in fluid-phase endocytosis, which appears to be mediated mainly by activation of the Ras pathway, is a compensatory response to the translocation of a population of intracellular vesicles to the cell surface after RTK activation (Wiley and Kaplan 1984; Bretscher and Aguado-Velasco 1998). It is clear that movement of membrane compartments is part of the biological response to growth factor stimulation. However, there still is no clear evidence to indicate that these processes are linked to the trafficking of the growth factor receptors themselves (Wiley and Kaplan 1984; Bretscher and Aguado-Velasco 1998; Wiley 1988; West et al. 1989).

Although degradation is the ultimate fate of internalized signal transducing receptors, the rate of receptor degradation is much slower than the rate of their internalization. It follows that substantial intracellular pools of receptors and ligands can accumulate on intracellular vesicles (Wiley et al. 1985). Although receptors are initially activated at the plasma membrane, activated receptors are also found on intracellular structures, notably endosomes. What remains unclear is the degree to which internalized receptors remain active before their degradation. Some of the strongest evidence supporting the "signaling endosome" hypothesis comes from recent genetic, morphological, and biochemical experiments with the EGF receptor and the adrenergic receptor. Vieira and colleagues (Vieira et al. 1996) used a conditional dynamin mutant to block EGF receptor endocytosis, resulting in specific signal transduction pathways being upregulated and others being attenuated. In similar experiments with the adrenergic receptor, using both dynamin and β-arrestin mutants inhibited endocytosis, which resulted in inhibition of Erk1/2 activation (Ahn et al. 1999; Daaka et al. 1998). Early experiments in rat hepatocytes demonstrated that after the administration of EGF, endosomal EGF receptor is associated with SH2 domain-containing transforming protein (Shc), growth factor receptor-bound protein 2 (Grb2), c-Src, and mSOS (Wiley et al. 1985; Di Guglielmo et al. 1994). These cofactors are thought to be responsible for initiating signals at the cell surface (van der Geer et al. 1994; Adamson et al. 1992; Kaplan et al. 1992).

Besides RTKs, there are other receptors that exhibit a link between signal transduction and endocytosis . Both endocytosis and signaling of G protein-coupled receptors (GPCRs) are regulated through interactions with the scaffolding protein β-arrestin, and through G protein α- and $\beta\gamma$ subunits, respectively. The β-arrestin proteins function as an adaptor that promotes the association of signaling factors with GPCRs. For example, they recruit Src to the β_2-adrenergic receptor (β_2AR), thus triggering tyrosine kinase activity (Luttrell et al. 1999). Similar recruitment of Src family kinases has been observed for several other GPCRs. Activated GPCRs are desensitized by phosphorylation and subsequent β-arrestin binding, which accelerates endocytosis of receptors and prevents further interaction with G protein effectors. The recruitment of GPCRs to clathrin-coated pits is aided by the interaction of the clathrin adaptor protein AP-2 with β-arrestin, and endocytosis is mediated by a direct β-arrestin-clathrin interaction (Laporte et al. 1999; Ferguson 2001; McDonald and Lefkowitz 2001; Laporte et al. 2002; Luttrell and Lefkowitz 2002).

The function of β-arrestin is not limited to regulating membrane trafficking of GPCRs. β-arrestins have been shown to be necessary for activation of the mitogen-activated protein kinase (MAPK) pathway by internalized receptors (McDonald and Lefkowitz 2001). Thus β-arrestins may play a central role in triggering a second wave of intracellular signaling by forming a scaffolding complex consisting of a number of different signaling molecules. Ligands for GPCRs are capable of activating mitogenic RTKs, in addition to the MAPK signaling pathway and classic G protein-dependent signaling pathways involving adenylyl cyclase and phospholipase. Many examples of transactivation of growth factor receptors in response to GPCR signaling have now been reported. In each case, dimerization and tyrosine phosphorylation of RTKs occur, followed by association of receptors with tyrosine phosphorylated adaptor proteins and Ras-dependent activation of MAPKs (McPherson et al. 2001; Luttrell et al. 1997; Hackel et al. 1999). A variety of diverse ligands for GPCRs have been observed to rapidly increase EGF receptor autophosphorylation. These include isoproterenol, thrombin, lysophosphatidic acid (LPA), endothelin, thyrotropin-releasing hormone, carbachol, and angiotensin II (Daub et al. 1996; Daub et al. 1997; Zwick et al. 1999). Recently, it has been shown that Trk RTKs (TrkA, TrkB, and TrkC) can also be activated via a GPCR mechanism, without involvement of neurotrophins (Lee and Chao 2001; Ralevic and Burnstock 1998). Adenosine and adenosine agonists can activate Trk receptor phosphorylation specifically through the seven transmembrane spanning adenosine 2A (A2A) receptor. Several features of Trk receptor transactivation are significantly different from other transactivation events (Berg et al. 1992; Zwick et al. 1999; Eguchi et al. 1998). Trk receptor transactivation is slower and results in a selective increase in activation of Akt. Therefore, GPCRs and RTKs can specifically activate both Akt and Erk1/2 kinase signaling. Furthermore, it has been discovered that Gα (Gα_s and Gα_i) can directly stimulate Src family tyrosine kinase activity (Gao et al. 1999; Seidel et al. 1999; Sexl et al. 1997). This novel regulation of Src tyrosine kinase by G proteins provides insights into the adenylyl cyclase-independent signaling mechanisms involved in ligand-induced receptor desensitization, internalization, and other physiological processes. Rab GTPases have also been shown to be intimately involved with the signaling response to GPCR activation and internalization (Seachrist et al. 2002; Seachrist and Ferguson 2003).

Another class of cell surface receptors consisting of the TGF-β receptor family also shows a link between endocytosis and signaling. In experiments that looked at the phosphorylation of Smad2 and its subsequent nuclear translocation as a readout for TGF-β signaling, inhibition of SARA localization to the endosome aborts signal propagation. SARA is a docking site for Smad found in endosomes and is upstream of Smad activation in the TGF-β signaling cascade (Hayes et al. 2002).

4
Signaling in Endosomes

Despite evidence to the contrary, it has been argued that EGF receptor signal transduction is primarily restricted to the cell surface (Di Fiore and Gill 1999). To a large extent, this idea is based on the correlation between low rates of EGF receptor internalization and cell transformation (Sexl et al. 1997; Han and Colicelli 1995). Supporting this argument is the observation that a EGF receptor mutant—C:973, which does not internalize or internalizes poorly—promotes cell transformation. The same reasoning would apply to v-Cbl-transformed cells, in which internalized EGF receptor might be rapidly recycled back to the cell surface (Wells et al. 1990; Levkowitz et al. 1998). Signaling through the phospholipase C-γ (PLC-γ) and phosphatidyinositol-3 (PI-3) kinase pathways appears to be limited to the cell surface, whereas signaling through the Ras pathway seems to occur throughout the intracellular itinerary of the activated RTK (Haugh et al. 1999; Haugh and Meyer 2002). These data suggest not only that signaling can arise from endosomes, but also that receptor trafficking can modulate both the specificity and the duration of the signal transduction process.

Rin1 has been identified as a novel Rab5 GEF (Tall et al. 2001). Rin1 was initially identified based on its ability to block Ras-induced cell death (Han and Colicelli 1995) and was also found in both plasma membrane and endosomes (Barbieri et al. 2003). Rin1 can also bind BCR-ABL and 14-3-3 proteins, as well as activated Ras (Lim et al. 2000; Afar et al. 1997; Han et al. 1997). Sequence analysis of Rin1 reveals the presence of several domains: an SH2 and a proline-rich domain in the amino-terminal region and a Ras-binding domain (RBD) in the carboxyl-terminal region. Work in our laboratory indicates that Rin1 contains a region (aa 443–569) that is homologous to the catalytic domain of the Vps9p-like Rab5 GEF (Tall et al. 2001). We also found that the SH2 region is necessary and sufficient for interaction with the EGF receptor cytoplasmic tail (Barbieri et al. 2003). Expression of Rin1 not only alters EGF receptor internalization but also affects EGF receptor stimulation of Raf and the activation of the Erk pathway. Surprisingly, the expression of Rin1-WT does not affect the activation of Ras, which suggests that Rin1 inhibits activation of the MAPK pathway through its RBD. Interestingly, Ras and EGF receptor localize with both Rin1 and Rab5 on "enlarged" early endosomes. (Roberts et al. 1999). These observations indicate that endosomes enriched in signaling proteins such as EGF receptor, Ras, PI3-kinase, Rin1, and Rab5 may constitute a platform for the generation of specific and unique signals. Consistent with this idea, fluid-phase endocytosis in A431 cells is increased by stimulation of EGF receptors, resulting in enlarged endocytic vesicles (Wiley and Cunningham 1982; Wells et al. 1990), and this appears to be due at least in part to the activation of Rab5 (Barbieri et al. 2000). Similarly, expression of constitutively active mutants of p21Ras is accompanied by increased endocytosis (Barbieri et al. 2001; Bar-Sagi and Feramisco 1986), and this effect is mediated by Rab5 (Barbieri et al. 2000; Tall et al. 2001). Overexpression of a Rab5a exchange factor, which would be expected to increase Rab5a-GTP levels, increases the rate of EGF receptor endocytosis. Rin1 is distinct from the previously described Rab5a exchange factor, Rabex-5 (Tall et al. 2001; Horiuchi et al. 1997). Recently, the stress-activated p38 kinase was shown to phosphorylate Rab-GDI, thereby increasing its ability to bind Rab5-GDP (Cavalli et al. 2001). With phosphorylated RabGDI, Rab5 is thought to be more efficiently recycled to the cytosol for subsequent delivery to endosomal membranes. Thus endocytosis is accelerated after stress (e.g., H_2O_2 exposure), and this acceleration is not observed in cells lacking p38 kinase.

The high level of activated EGF receptor found in endosomes is a direct result of ligand-induced endocytosis ; however, the situation with other ErbB family members may vary. Although ErbB2–3 exhibit significantly slower internalization rates, the effective signaling time period may not necessarily be longer, because of their more rapid and constitutive targeting to the lysosomes (Oksvold et al. 2001). Thus, in the case of EGF receptor signaling, endosomes represent the primary signaling compartment, whereas the cell surface represents the primary compartment for the other members of the ErbB family.

Late endosomes may also play a key role in signaling responses to growth factors and stress (e.g., starvation). Availability of extracellular nutrients to cells exerts a constitutive control over entry and exit from the cell cycle. There is evidence to suggest that this control is mediated by Rab7 through its effect on the endosome-lysosome pathway (Edinger et al. 2003).

RTK-mediated signal transduction is accomplished by multiple phases of protein–protein interactions. The first phase consists of proteins that directly bind to activated receptors. These adaptor proteins recognize receptor phosphotyrosines through their SH2 and PTB domains. Several receptor-interacting proteins are found in endosomes, which is consistent with the persistence of a phosphorylated state for internalized receptors (Fig. 2). For example, growth factor receptor-bound protein 2 (Grb2) and SH2 domain-containing transforming protein (Shc) adaptors are readily detected in endosomes that contain activated EGF receptors (Joneson and Bar-Sagi 1997; Choy et al. 1999). Recruitment of Grb2 to the membrane by direct interaction with receptors or indirectly through Shc, fibroblast growth factor receptor substrate (FRS), or insulin receptor substrate (IRS) adaptors is the key event in activation of the small GTPase Ras (Schlessinger 2000). Because Grb2 is constitutively associated with son-of-sevenless (SOS), a Ras GEF, the proximity of Grb2-SOS complexes and Ras at the membrane elevates GTP loading of Ras.

Ras-GTPases have crucial roles in RTK signaling. Ras-GTP loading is thought to be necessary for activation of several signaling pathways (Joneson and Bar-Sagi 1997). Ras is found at the plasma membrane and in intracellular membranes, including those of endosomes (Choy et al. 1999; Rizzo et al. 2000; Rizzo et al. 2001; Jiang and Sorkin 2002). In some cells Ras is constitutively associated with endosomes, whereas in other cells Ras is internalized from the cell surface in response to stimulation. If Grb2-SOS complexes activate Ras at the plasma membrane, what would be the role of Ras localization and activity in endosomes? An important consideration might be the localization of Ras relative to the distribution of its regulators and effectors. The accumulation of Grb2-SOS complexes in endosomes might serve to sustain Ras activity for a prolonged time. The serine/threonine kinase c-Raf-1, an important effector of Ras, is also translocated to endosomes in response to receptor activation (Choy et al. 1999; Rizzo et al. 2000; Rizzo et al. 2001; Jiang and Sorkin 2002). Another putative effector of Ras, Rab5, is a resident protein of the early endosomal compartment (Barbieri et al. 2000). By contrast, RTK-activated enzymes such as PLC1γ and PI-3 kinase, which localize to endosomes, are spatially separated from their substrate—phosphatidylinositol 4,5-bisphosphate—which is mainly located at the plasma membrane (Haugh et al. 1999; Haugh and Meyer 2002; Barbieri et al. 2001). Furthermore, Erk and Mek kinases, which function downstream of Raf, have also been detected biochemically in purified endosomal fractions and localized to endosomes by immunofluorescence microscopy (Barbieri et al. 2000; Haugh and Meyer 2002;). Recruitment of these kinases to endosomes is presumably mediated by kinase-substrate inter-

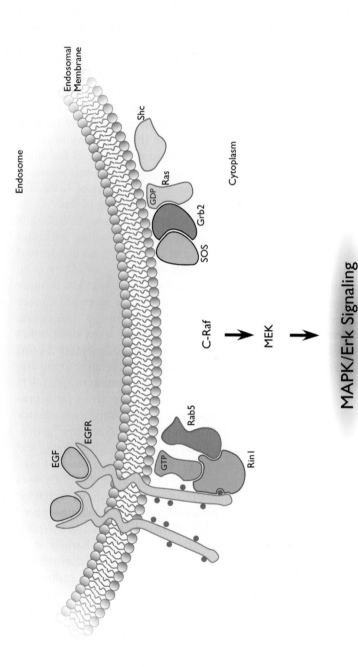

Fig. 2. Signaling from endosomes: This model for a signaling cascade originating from endosomes uses EGF receptor as an example. After binding of EGF to the receptor at the cell surface, it is autophosphorylated and internalized. The phosphorylated state of the receptor persists in the endosome. The activated receptor then forms a complex with Rin1, Rab5a, and Ras-GTP. The Ras is activated and recruited to the endosome by Shc, Grb2, and SOS. The GTP-loaded Ras then recruits C-Raf to the endosome, which in turn activates MEK, thus initiating the MAPK/Erk pathway

actions, Erk/MAPK scaffolds, and/or unidentified membrane proteins (Haugh and Meyer 2002; Wunderlich et al. 2001).

Similar to Ras, the GTPase Rap can also be copurified with endosomes that contain activated TrkA receptors (Wu et al. 2001). With a coimmunoprecipitation assay, Rap1 was found to associate with activated TrkA receptors, the adaptors CrkL and Grb2-associated binding protein 2 (Gab2), C3G (an exchange factor for Rap1), B-Raf, activated Mek, and Erk1/2. Maintenance of Rap1 signaling complexes in endosomes might serve to sustain Rap1 and Erk1/2 activity in neuronal cells, which is important for neuronal differentiation (Wu et al. 2001; York et al. 1998).

5
Sorting in Endosomes

The second key stage of endocytic transport of signaling receptors is their sorting in endosomes. Endocytic sorting involves highly specific mechanisms that can sort distinct receptors with high efficiency to either divergent recycling or degradative pathways within several minutes of coendocytosis. The predominant model proposes that internalized receptors are prevented from recycling by becoming sequestered inside MVEs (Fig. 1). This model is based mainly on studies of differential sorting of EGF and transferrin receptors in mammalian cells and, more recently, on the studies of protein sorting in yeast (Hopkins 1992; Katzmann et al. 2001). The correlation of ubiquitylation, interaction with ubiquitin ligases, and degradation rates of RTKs and GPCRs indicates that ubiquitylation of cytoplasmic lysine residues might be important for the retention and sequestration of these receptors in MVEs (Marchese and Benovic 2001; Peschard et al. 2001; Shenoy et al. 2001). Recent studies in yeast indicate that ubiquitylation might promote sorting of several membrane proteins to the yeast vacuole through the interaction of ubiquitylated proteins with a protein complex that contains vacuole protein sorting gene 23 (Vps23) (Marchese and Benovic 2001). Recent studies have demonstrated a strong correlation between c-Cbl-mediated ubiquitylation of the EGF receptor and accelerated degradation (Levkowitz et al. 1998). c-Cbl functions as an ubiquitin-protein ligase, or E3 (Shenoy et al. 2001; Levkowitz et al. 1999; Yokouchi et al. 1999; Jongeward et al. 1995). Expression of the truncated form of c-Cbl also regulates platelet-derived growth factor (PDGF) and colony-stimulating factor-1 (CSF-1) receptors (Miyake et al. 1999; Lee et al. 1999). It has been suggested that c-Cbl is the primary regulator of EGF receptor trafficking between early and late endosomes (Levkowitz et al. 1999), but this seems unlikely for a number of reasons. First, the activity of c-Cbl requires receptor kinase activity and phosphorylation at residue 1045 (Levkowitz et al. 1999). However, numerous studies have shown that endosomal sorting and lysosomal targeting do not require receptor kinase activity (French et al. 1994; Wiley et al. 1991; Herbst et al. 1994). Furthermore, EGF receptors truncated to residue 1022, which lack a c-Cbl binding site, are internalized and degraded at a rate indistinguishable from that of full-length receptors. In addition, a c-Cbl-associated protein "sprouty" acts as a positive regulator of EGF signaling (Murphy et al. 1998).

Even though c-Cbl is unlikely to be an obligatory component of the endocytic sorting machinery, it does appear to be an important regulator of activated RTKs. Knockout mice lacking c-Cbl show hyperproliferation and excess branching in the mammary epithelium, as would be expected of a negative regulator of intracellular EGF receptor pools (Wiley et al. 1991). Overexpression of c-Cbl significantly stimulates the ligand-induced degradation of EGF and PDGF receptors, and truncated forms of Cbl can also act as dominant-negative inhibitors of EGF receptor sorting (Levkowitz et al. 1998). This indicates that c-Cbl interacts with receptor sites crucial for normal receptor trafficking. Although RTK activity is not required for lysosomal targeting of the EGF receptor, it can significantly enhance the sorting of full-length receptors (Waterman et al. 1998), consistent with a role for c-Cbl as a modulator of EGF receptor degradation. A model compatible with most current data is that c-Cbl binds to kinase-active EGF receptor, mediates receptor ubiquitylation, and then dissociates. Ubiquitin functions as a receptor "tag" that increases receptor affinity for the lysosomal targeting machinery or stimulates vesiculation of MVEs, resulting in enhanced receptor degradation (Katzmann et al. 2001). The degradation of ubiquitylated receptors is thought to occur more through the lysosomal pathway and less via the proteasome-mediated pathway (Levkowitz et al. 1999). Although certain receptors, such as c-Met (Hammond et al. 2001), are degraded via the proteasome pathway, the preference for the lysosomal pathway is due to the presence of ligand-induced multiple monoubiquitin moieties as opposed to polyubiquitin chains (Pickart 2001; Hicke 2001; Weissman 2001; Haglund et al. 2003).

Studies of a class of yeast vacuolar protein sorting (*vps*) mutants that have endosomal trafficking defects have provided insight into the cargo selection machinery. A strong candidate for the cargo receptor that recognizes the ubiquitin tag (Katzmann et al. 2003) is endosomal sorting complex required for transport (ESCRT-I), a conserved 350-kDa complex consisting of the E Vps proteins Vps23, Vps28, and Vps37. ESCRT-I binds ubiquitin in vitro and ubiquitylated cargo in vivo. Although these interactions may be indirect, they do require the Vps23p presumed ubiquitin-binding domain. Mutation of this domain not only prevents the sorting of ubiquitylated cargo into internal vesicles of MVEs but also prevents the formation of the vesicles themselves, suggesting that the recognition of cargo by ESCRT-I activates downstream components of the vesicle budding machinery. These downstream components are known as ESCRT II and III. Tumor susceptibility gene 101 (TSG101), the human ortholog of Vps23, has been found to have a prominent role in the sorting of proteins after internalization. Through its ability to bind ubiquitin, it is involved in the sorting of ubiquitylated proteins like RTKs to MVEs. Along with HRS, another ubiquitin binding protein that is involved in the sorting of internalized proteins in the early endosome, TSG101 plays a role in signal transduction from endocytosed RTKs by determining their trafficking fate. Interestingly, HRS and TSG101 have been shown to interact with each other to add another level of complexity to the sorting process (Lu et al. 2003).

Recently, a number of publications have suggested that ubiquitylation is necessary for internalization of the EGF receptor (Wong et al. 2002; Soubeyran et al. 2002). Although these reports are of interest, they are far from definitive and are inconsistent with much of the current literature. For example, receptor domains that are required for c-Cbl binding and ubiquitylation can be removed from EGF receptor without significantly altering the rate of endocytosis (Wiley et al. 1991). However, endocytosis does not directly measure EGFR infernadization. Measuring EGF receptor loss or redistribution as opposed to internalization may yield variable results. Overexpression of potent regulatory molecules also complicates the interpretation of these studies. Furthermore, disruption of the dynamics of EGF receptor docking proteins can have unrelated secondary consequences.

6
A Perspective on Signaling Endosomes

It is clear that endocytosis and signaling are linked in important ways. Understanding how interactions between receptors and intracellular signaling molecules such as adaptors, GTPases, and kinases are regulated in intact cells will undoubtedly provide insight into the ways that cells sense and adapt to environmental conditions.

Remodeling of the cell surface, movement of endocytic organelles, and reorganization of the cytoskeleton on RTK stimulation may confer precise control of location, duration, and specificity to different signal transduction pathways. Internalized receptors may signal from sorting endosomes, recycling endosomes, or intermediate compartments such as transport vesicles or tubules. Thus the endomembrane system constitutes the most extensive membrane platform present in eukaryotic cells. We speculate that this membrane platform creates the opportunity for greater diversity of signals than can be generated from a limited number of molecules functioning in a single location.

Finally, an understanding of the molecular mechanisms of signal generation at the subcellular level, particularly when compartment-specific pathways are involved, might also offer new targets for therapeutics designed to block one but not all outputs from a particular signaling module.

While this review was in preparation, Miacynska et al. (2004) published work on APPL, a molecule involved in linking EGF receptor, Rab5 and transcription.

Acknowledgments We thank D. Owyoung for editing assistance. This work was supported in part by grants from the National Institutes of Health (GM-42259, AI-35884, and AI-20015 to P.D.S.) and from the Jose Carreras International Leukemia Foundation, Washington University's Siteman Cancer Center and Diabetes Research and Training Center (E.D. Thomas Fellowship Program, IRG5801045–1 and 2P60DK20579 to M.A.B.).

References

Adamson, P., H.F. Paterson, and A. Hall, Intracellular localization of the P21rho proteins. J Cell Biol, 1992. 119(3): p. 617–27

Afar, D.E., et al. Regulation of the oncogenic activity of BCR-ABL by a tightly bound substrate protein RIN1. Immunity, 1997. 6(6): p. 773–82

Ahn, S., et al. Src-mediated tyrosine phosphorylation of dynamin is required for beta2-adrenergic receptor internalization and mitogen-activated protein kinase signaling. J Biol Chem, 1999. 274(3): p. 1185–8

Barbieri, M.A., et al. Epidermal growth factor and membrane trafficking. EGF receptor activation of endocytosis requires Rab5a. J Cell Biol, 2000. 151(3): p. 539–50

Barbieri, M.A., et al. Phosphatidylinositol-4-phosphate 5-kinase-1beta is essential for epidermal growth factor receptor-mediated endocytosis. J Biol Chem, 2001. 276(50): p. 47212–6

Barbieri, M.A., et al. The SRC homology 2 domain of Rin1 mediates its binding to the epidermal growth factor receptor and regulates receptor endocytosis. J Biol Chem, 2003. 278(34): p. 32027–36

Bar-Sagi, D. and J.R. Feramisco, Induction of membrane ruffling and fluid-phase pinocytosis in quiescent fibroblasts by ras proteins. Science, 1986. 233(4768): p. 1061–8

Berg, M.M., et al. K-252a inhibits nerve growth factor-induced trk proto-oncogene tyrosine phosphorylation and kinase activity. J Biol Chem, 1992. 267(1): p. 13–6

Bretscher, M.S. and C. Aguado-Velasco, EGF induces recycling membrane to form ruffles. Curr Biol, 1998. 8(12): p. 721–4

Carbone, R., et al. Eps15 and eps15R are essential components of the endocytic pathway. Cancer Res, 1997. 57(24): p. 5498–504

Carpentier, J.L., et al. Co-localization of 125I-epidermal growth factor and ferritin-low density lipoprotein in coated pits: a quantitative electron microscopic study in normal and mutant human fibroblasts. J Cell Biol, 1982. 95(1): p. 73–7

Cavalli, V., et al. The stress-induced MAP kinase p38 regulates endocytic trafficking via the GDI:Rab5 complex. Mol Cell, 2001. 7(2): p. 421–32

Choy, E., et al. Endomembrane trafficking of ras: the CAAX motif targets proteins to the ER and Golgi. Cell, 1999. 98(1): p. 69–80

Daaka, Y., et al. Essential role for G protein-coupled receptor endocytosis in the activation of mitogen-activated protein kinase. J Biol Chem, 1998. 273(2): p. 685–8

Damke, H., et al. Induction of mutant dynamin specifically blocks endocytic coated vesicle formation. J Cell Biol, 1994. 127(4): p. 915–34

Daub, H., et al. Role of transactivation of the EGF receptor in signalling by G-protein-coupled receptors. Nature, 1996. 379(6565): p. 557–60

Daub, H., et al. Signal characteristics of G protein-transactivated EGF receptor. EMBO J, 1997. 16(23): p. 7032–44

Di Fiore, P.P. and G.N. Gill, Endocytosis and mitogenic signaling. Curr Opin Cell Biol, 1999. 11(4): p. 483–8

Di Guglielmo, G.M., et al. Compartmentalization of SHC, GRB2 and mSOS, and hyperphosphorylation of Raf-1 by EGF but not insulin in liver parenchyma. EMBO J, 1994. 13(18): p. 4269–77

Edinger, A.L., R.M. Cinalli, and C.B. Thompson, Rab7 prevents growth factor-independent survival by inhibiting cell-autonomous nutrient transporter expression. Dev Cell, 2003. 5(4): p. 571–82

Eguchi, S., et al. Calcium-dependent epidermal growth factor receptor transactivation mediates the angiotensin II-induced mitogen-activated protein kinase activation in vascular smooth muscle cells. J Biol Chem, 1998. 273(15): p. 8890–6

Felder, S., et al. Kinase activity controls the sorting of the epidermal growth factor receptor within the multivesicular body. Cell, 1990. 61(4): p. 623–34

Ferguson, S.S., Evolving concepts in G protein-coupled receptor endocytosis: the role in receptor desensitization and signaling. Pharmacol Rev, 2001. 53(1): p. 1–24

French, A.R., et al. Postendocytic trafficking of epidermal growth factor-receptor complexes is mediated through saturable and specific endosomal interactions. J Biol Chem, 1994. 269(22): p. 15749–55

Gao, Z., et al. A2B adenosine and P2Y2 receptors stimulate mitogen-activated protein kinase in human embryonic kidney-293 cells. Cross-talk between cyclic AMP and protein kinase C pathways. J Biol Chem, 1999. 274(9): p. 5972–80

Gorden, P., et al. Epidermal growth factor: morphological demonstration of binding, internalization, and lysosomal association in human fibroblasts. Proc Natl Acad Sci U S A, 1978. 75(10): p. 5025–9

Gruenberg, J. and F.R. Maxfield, Membrane transport in the endocytic pathway. Curr Opin Cell Biol, 1995. 7(4): p. 552–63

Hackel, P.O., et al. Epidermal growth factor receptors: critical mediators of multiple receptor pathways. Curr Opin Cell Biol, 1999. 11(2): p. 184–9

Haglund, K., P.P. Di Fiore, and I. Dikic, Distinct monoubiquitin signals in receptor endocytosis. Trends Biochem Sci, 2003. 28(11): p. 598–604

Haigler, H.T., J.A. McKanna, and S. Cohen, Rapid stimulation of pinocytosis in human carcinoma cells A-431 by epidermal growth factor. J Cell Biol, 1979. 83(1): p. 82–90

Hammond, D.E., et al. Down-regulation of MET, the receptor for hepatocyte growth factor. Oncogene, 2001. 20(22): p. 2761–70

Han, L. and J. Colicelli, A human protein selected for interference with Ras function interacts directly with Ras and competes with Raf1. Mol Cell Biol, 1995. 15(3): p. 1318–23

Han, L., et al. Protein binding and signaling properties of RIN1 suggest a unique effector function. Proc Natl Acad Sci U S A, 1997. 94(10): p. 4954–9

Hanover, J.A., M.C. Willingham, and I. Pastan, Kinetics of transit of transferrin and epidermal growth factor through clathrin-coated membranes. Cell, 1984. 39 (2 Pt 1): p. 283–93

Haugh, J.M., et al. Internalized epidermal growth factor receptors participate in the activation of p21(ras) in fibroblasts. J Biol Chem, 1999. 274(48): p. 34350–60

Haugh, J.M. and T. Meyer, Active EGF receptors have limited access to PtdIns(4,5)P(2) in endosomes: implications for phospholipase C and PI 3-kinase signaling. J Cell Sci, 2002. 115(Pt 2): p. 303–10

Hayes, S., A. Chawla, and S. Corvera, TGF beta receptor internalization into EEA1-enriched early endosomes: role in signaling to Smad2. J Cell Biol, 2002. 158(7): p. 1239–49

Herbst, J.J., et al. Regulation of postendocytic trafficking of the epidermal growth factor receptor through endosomal retention. J Biol Chem, 1994. 269(17): p. 12865–73

Hicke, L., Protein regulation by monoubiquitin. Nat Rev Mol Cell Biol, 2001. 2(3): p. 195–201

Hopkins, C.R., Selective membrane protein trafficking: vectorial flow and filter. Trends Biochem Sci, 1992. 17(1): p. 27–32

Hopkins, C.R., K. Miller, and J.M. Beardmore, Receptor-mediated endocytosis of transferrin and epidermal growth factor receptors: a comparison of constitutive and ligand-induced uptake. J Cell Sci Suppl, 1985. 3: p. 173–86

Horiuchi, H., et al. A novel Rab5 GDP/GTP exchange factor complexed to Rabaptin-5 links nucleotide exchange to effector recruitment and function. Cell, 1997. 90(6): p. 1149–59

Jiang, X. and A. Sorkin, Coordinated traffic of Grb2 and Ras during epidermal growth factor receptor endocytosis visualized in living cells. Mol Biol Cell, 2002. 13(5): p. 1522–35

Joneson, T. and D. Bar-Sagi, Ras effectors and their role in mitogenesis and oncogenesis. J Mol Med, 1997. 75(8): p. 587–93

Jongeward, G.D., T.R. Clandinin, and P.W. Sternberg, sli-1, a negative regulator of let-23-mediated signaling in C. elegans. Genetics, 1995. 139(4): p. 1553–66

Kaplan, K.B., et al. Association of p60c-src with endosomal membranes in mammalian fibroblasts. J Cell Biol, 1992. 118(2): p. 321–33

Katzmann, D.J., M. Babst, and S.D. Emr, Ubiquitin-dependent sorting into the multivesicular body pathway requires the function of a conserved endosomal protein sorting complex, ESCRT-I. Cell, 2001. 106(2): p. 145–55

Katzmann, D.J., et al. Vps27 recruits ESCRT machinery to endosomes during MVB sorting. J Cell Biol, 2003. 162(3): p. 413–23

Laporte, S.A., et al. The beta2-adrenergic receptor/betaarrestin complex recruits the clathrin adaptor AP-2 during endocytosis. Proc Natl Acad Sci U S A, 1999. 96(7): p. 3712–7

Laporte, S.A., et al. beta-Arrestin/AP-2 interaction in G protein-coupled receptor internalization: identification of a beta-arrestin binging site in beta 2-adaptin. J Biol Chem, 2002. 277(11): p. 9247–54

Lee, F.S. and M.V. Chao, Activation of Trk neurotrophin receptors in the absence of neurotrophins. Proc Natl Acad Sci U S A, 2001. 98(6): p. 3555–60

Lee, P.S., et al. The Cbl protooncoprotein stimulates CSF-1 receptor multiubiquitination and endocytosis, and attenuates macrophage proliferation. EMBO J, 1999. 18(13): p. 3616–28

Levkowitz, G., et al. c-Cbl/Sli-1 regulates endocytic sorting and ubiquitination of the epidermal growth factor receptor. Genes Dev, 1998. 12(23): p. 3663–74

Levkowitz, G., et al. Ubiquitin ligase activity and tyrosine phosphorylation underlie suppression of growth factor signaling by c-Cbl/Sli-1. Mol Cell, 1999. 4(6): p. 1029–40

Lim, Y.M., et al. BCR/ABL inhibition by an escort/phosphatase fusion protein. Proc Natl Acad Sci U S A, 2000. 97(22): p. 12233–8

Lu, Q., et al. TSG101 interaction with HRS mediates endosomal trafficking and receptor down-regulation. Proc Natl Acad Sci U S A, 2003. 100(13): p. 7626–31

Luttrell, L.M., et al. Gbetagamma subunits mediate Src-dependent phosphorylation of the epidermal growth factor receptor. A scaffold for G protein-coupled receptor-mediated Ras activation. J Biol Chem, 1997. 272(7): p. 4637–44

Luttrell, L.M., et al. Beta-arrestin-dependent formation of beta2 adrenergic receptor-Src protein kinase complexes. Science, 1999. 283(5402): p. 655–61

Luttrell, L.M. and R.J. Lefkowitz, The role of beta-arrestins in the termination and transduction of G-protein-coupled receptor signals. J Cell Sci, 2002. 115(Pt 3): p. 455–65

Marchese, A. and J.L. Benovic, Agonist-promoted ubiquitination of the G protein-coupled receptor CXCR4 mediates lysosomal sorting. J Biol Chem, 2001. 276(49): p. 45509–12

McDonald, P.H. and R.J. Lefkowitz, Beta-Arrestins: new roles in regulating heptahelical receptors' functions. Cell Signal, 2001. 13(10): p. 683–9

McKanna, J.A., H.T. Haigler, and S. Cohen, Hormone receptor topology and dynamics: morphological analysis using ferritin-labeled epidermal growth factor. Proc Natl Acad Sci U S A, 1979. 76(11): p. 5689–93

McPherson, P.S., B.K. Kay, and N.K. Hussain, Signaling on the endocytic pathway. Traffic, 2001. 2(6): p. 375–84

Mesa, R., et al. Rab22a affects the morphology and function of the endocytic pathway. J Cell Sci, 2001. 114(Pt 22): p. 4041–4049

Miacynska, M., et al. APPL proteins link Rab5 to nuclear signal transducion via an endosomal compartment. Cell, 2004. 116(2): p. 445–456

Miller, K., et al. Localization of the epidermal growth factor (EGF) receptor within the endosome of EGF-stimulated epidermoid carcinoma (A431) cells. J Cell Biol, 1986. 102(2): p. 500–9

Miyake, S., et al. Cbl-mediated negative regulation of platelet-derived growth factor receptor-dependent cell proliferation. A critical role for Cbl tyrosine kinase-binding domain. J Biol Chem, 1999. 274(23): p. 16619–28

Murphy, M.A., et al. Tissue hyperplasia and enhanced T-cell signalling via ZAP-70 in c-Cbl-deficient mice. Mol Cell Biol, 1998. 18(8): p. 4872–82

Neer, E.J., Heterotrimeric G proteins: organizers of transmembrane signals. Cell, 1995. 80(2): p. 249–57

Oksvold, M.P., et al. Re-localization of activated EGF receptor and its signal transducers to multivesicular compartments downstream of early endosomes in response to EGF. Eur J Cell Biol, 2001. 80(4): p. 285–94

Peschard, P., et al. Mutation of the c-Cbl TKB domain binding site on the Met receptor tyrosine kinase converts it into a transforming protein. Mol Cell, 2001. 8(5): p. 995–1004

Pickart, C.M., Mechanisms underlying ubiquitination. Annu Rev Biochem, 2001. 70: p. 503–33

Ralevic, V. and G. Burnstock, Receptors for purines and pyrimidines. Pharmacol Rev, 1998. 50(3): p. 413–92

Rizzo, M.A., et al. The recruitment of Raf-1 to membranes is mediated by direct interaction with phosphatidic acid and is independent of association with Ras. J Biol Chem, 2000. 275(31): p. 23911–8

Rizzo, M.A., et al. Agonist-dependent traffic of raft-associated Ras and Raf-1 is required for activation of the mitogen-activated protein kinase cascade. J Biol Chem, 2001. 276(37): p. 34928–33

Roberts, R.L., et al. Endosome fusion in living cells overexpressing GFP-rab5. J Cell Sci, 1999. 112 (Pt 21): p. 3667–75

Schlessinger, J., Cell signaling by receptor tyrosine kinases. Cell, 2000. 103(2): p. 211–25

Seachrist, J.L., et al. Rab5 association with the angiotensin II type 1A receptor promotes Rab5 GTP binding and vesicular fusion. J Biol Chem, 2002. 277(1): p. 679–85

Seachrist, J.L. and S.S. Ferguson, Regulation of G protein-coupled receptor endocytosis and trafficking by Rab GTPases. Life Sci, 2003. 74(2–3): p. 225–35

Seidel, M.G., et al. Activation of mitogen-activated protein kinase by the A_{2A}-adenosine receptor via a rap1-dependent and via a p21(ras)-dependent pathway. J Biol Chem, 1999. 274(36): p. 25833–41

Sexl, V., et al. Stimulation of the mitogen-activated protein kinase via the A2A-adenosine receptor in primary human endothelial cells. J Biol Chem, 1997. 272(9): p. 5792–9

Shenoy, S.K., et al. Regulation of receptor fate by ubiquitination of activated beta 2-adrenergic receptor and beta-arrestin. Science, 2001. 294(5545): p. 1307–13

Sorkin, A., et al. Recycling of epidermal growth factor-receptor complexes in A431 cells: identification of dual pathways. J Cell Biol, 1991. 112(1): p. 55–63

Soubeyran, P., et al. Cbl-CIN85-endophilin complex mediates ligand-induced downregulation of EGF receptors. Nature, 2002. 416(6877): p. 183–7

Tall, G.G., et al. Ras-activated endocytosis is mediated by the Rab5 guanine nucleotide exchange activity of RIN1. Dev Cell, 2001. 1(1): p. 73–82

van der Geer, P., T. Hunter, and R.A. Lindberg, Receptor protein-tyrosine kinases and their signal transduction pathways. Annu Rev Cell Biol, 1994. 10: p. 251–337

Vieira, A.V., C. Lamaze, and S.L. Schmid, Control of EGF receptor signaling by clathrin-mediated endocytosis. Science, 1996. 274(5295): p. 2086–9

Waterman, H., et al. Alternative intracellular routing of ErbB receptors may determine signaling potency. J Biol Chem, 1998. 273(22): p. 13819–27

Weissman, A.M., Themes and variations on ubiquitylation. Nat Rev Mol Cell Biol, 2001. 2(3): p. 169–78

Wells, A., et al. Ligand-induced transformation by a noninternalizing epidermal growth factor receptor. Science, 1990. 247(4945): p. 962–4

West, M.A., M.S. Bretscher, and C. Watts, Distinct endocytotic pathways in epidermal growth factor-stimulated human carcinoma A431 cells. J Cell Biol, 1989. 109(6 Pt 1): p. 2731–9

Wiley, H.S., Anomalous binding of epidermal growth factor to A431 cells is due to the effect of high receptor densities and a saturable endocytic system. J Cell Biol, 1988. 107(2): p. 801–10

Wiley, H.S. and D.D. Cunningham, Epidermal growth factor stimulates fluid phase endocytosis in human fibroblasts through a signal generated at the cell surface. J Cell Biochem, 1982. 19(4): p. 383–94

Wiley, H.S. and J. Kaplan, Epidermal growth factor rapidly induces a redistribution of transferrin receptor pools in human fibroblasts. Proc Natl Acad Sci U S A, 1984. 81(23): p. 7456–60

Wiley, H.S., et al. Intracellular processing of epidermal growth factor and its effect on ligand-receptor interactions. J Biol Chem, 1985. 260(9): p. 5290–5

Wiley, H.S., et al. The role of tyrosine kinase activity in endocytosis, compartmentation, and down-regulation of the epidermal growth factor receptor. J Biol Chem, 1991. 266(17): p. 11083–94

Wong, E.S., et al. Sprouty2 attenuates epidermal growth factor receptor ubiquitylation and endocytosis, and consequently enhances Ras/ERK signalling. EMBO J, 2002. 21(18): p. 4796–808

Wu, C., C.F. Lai, and W.C. Mobley, Nerve growth factor activates persistent Rap1 signaling in endosomes. J Neurosci, 2001. 21(15): p. 5406–16

Wunderlich, W., et al. A novel 14-kilodalton protein interacts with the mitogen-activated protein kinase scaffold mp1 on a late endosomal/lysosomal compartment. J Cell Biol, 2001. 152(4): p. 765–76

Yokouchi, M., et al. Ligand-induced ubiquitination of the epidermal growth factor receptor involves the interaction of the c-Cbl RING finger and UbcH7. J Biol Chem, 1999. 274(44): p. 31707–12

York, R.D., et al. Rap1 mediates sustained MAP kinase activation induced by nerve growth factor. Nature, 1998. 392(6676): p. 622–6

Zwick, E., et al. Distinct calcium-dependent pathways of epidermal growth factor receptor transactivation and PYK2 tyrosine phosphorylation in PC12 cells. J Biol Chem, 1999. 274(30): p. 20989–96

Zwick, E., et al. The EGF receptor as central transducer of heterologous signalling systems. Trends Pharmacol Sci, 1999. 20(10): p. 408–12

CTMI (2004) 286:21–44
© Springer-Verlag 2004

Met Receptor Dynamics and Signalling

D. E. Hammond · S. Carter · M. J. Clague (✉)

Physiological Laboratory, University of Liverpool, Crown Street, Liverpool,
L69 3BX, UK
clague@liv.ac.uk

Abstract The receptor for hepatocyte growth factor (HGF), Met, controls a programme of invasive growth that combines proliferation with various moto- and morphogenetic processes. This process is important for development and organ regeneration, but dysregulation in transformed tissues can contribute to cancer progression and metastasis. Acute stimulation of tissue culture cells with HGF leads to Met downregulation via degradation through an endocytic mechanism that also requires proteasome activity. Perturbation of Met trafficking on the endocytic pathway, either at the level of the internalisation step or during sorting at the early endosome, leads to altered signalling outputs. Ubiquitination of Met through the E3-ligase Cbl is required for receptor downregulation, and a mutant receptor defective in Cbl binding is able to transform cells. We discuss the hypothesis that some naturally occurring Met mutants implicated in cancer may transform cells owing to defects in their trafficking along the endosomal degradation pathway.

1
Background

1.1
The Hepatocyte Growth Factor-Met Receptor System

Hepatocyte growth factor (HGF) was originally identified as a powerful mitogen for hepatocytes in primary culture (Nakamura et al. 1984; Russell et al. 1984a; Russell et al. 1984b). It was later shown to be indistinguishable from scatter factor (SF), a secretory product of fibroblasts which dissociates epithelial cells and increases their motility and invasiveness (Naldini et al. 1991b; Stoker et al. 1987; Weidner et al. 1991). HGF is synthesised and secreted as a biologically inactive precursor (pro-HGF) and is activated through proteolytic cleavage (Naka et al. 1992) into a mature, disulphide-linked heterodimer consisting of a 69-kDa α-chain and a 34-kDa β-chain. Functional studies in the early 1990s identified HGF as the ligand for Met receptor (Bottaro et al. 1991; Naldini et al. 1991b; Rubin et al. 1991). The α-chain of HGF is responsible for binding to Met, and the β-chain is required for full receptor activation and execution of its biological responses (Matsumoto et al. 1998). HGF is produced mainly by cells of mesenchymal origin and interacts with Met receptors expressed on other cell types that do not express the ligand, typically epithelial and endothelial cells. This paracrine mechanism of action is a general and distinctive feature of the HGF-Met system.

Met receptor was first identified as the product of a human oncogene, *tpr-met*, which results from the chromosomal translocation and fusion of two distinct genetic loci: *tpr*, which contributes a protein-protein dimerisation motif; and *met*, which contributes the intracellular portion of the Met receptor. Molecular cloning indicated that the product of the

→

Fig. 1. The structure of Met and the signalling complex recruited to it on HGF stimulation and receptor dimerisation. Met is a single-pass disulphide-linked α/β heterodimer formed by proteolytic processing of a precursor in a post-Golgi compartment. The intracellular domain contains a tyrosine kinase catalytic region (*dark blue boxes*) flanked by distinctive juxtamembrane and C-terminal sequences. Signalling by the receptor is achieved through a multisubstrate docking site around Tyr[1349] and Tyr[1356] which mediates receptor interactions with multiple signal-transducing and adaptor proteins, including Gab1, Grb2/SOS, PI3-kinase and PLCγ. Such interactions are important for the generation of HGF-mediated invasive growth thought to play an essential role in a wide range of normal physiological processes (embryogenesis, tissue repair, angiogenesis etc.) as well as in tumour development and progression.

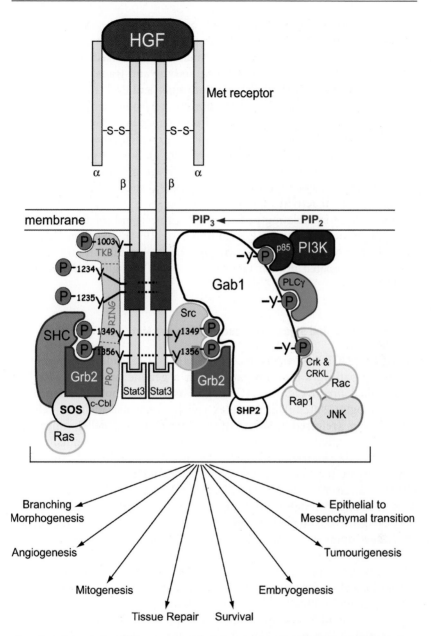

Phosphorylation of Tyr[1003] is responsible for recruiting the ubiquitin E3 ligase adaptor protein Cbl, leading to receptor ubiquitination and downregulation via degradation

entire Met gene had the characteristics of a cell surface growth factor receptor tyrosine kinase (RTK) (Dean et al. 1985; Park et al. 1987). The chimeric tpr-met fusion protein is permanently dimerised and activated, possessing constitutive tyrosine kinase activity and transforming ability (Cooper et al. 1984; Park et al. 1986; Rodrigues and Park 1993).

Met is a single-pass plasma membrane heterodimer of 190 kDa. It consists of a heavily glycosylated, entirely extracellular α-chain (50 kDa) and a membrane-spanning β-chain (140 kDa) which possesses intrinsic, ligand-activated tyrosine kinase activity (Fig. 1). Both α- and β-subunits are derived by intracellular proteolytic cleavage of a common 170-kDa single-chain precursor (Giordano et al. 1989), and both are necessary for the biological activity of Met.

Macrophage-stimulating protein (MSP), the ligand for the Ron RTK, is highly homologous to HGF (Gaudino et al. 1994). Together, HGF and MSP constitute a family of SFs with similar biological activities termed plasminogen-related growth factors (PRGFs) (Comoglio and Boccaccio 2001).

1.2
Invasive Growth and Signal Transduction Through Met

Binding of HGF to the Met receptor triggers a cascade of intracellular signalling pathways that ultimately elicit a genetic programme leading to so-called *invasive growth* (Comoglio and Trusolino 2002; Trusolino and Comoglio 2002). This complex cellular response includes cell-cell dissociation (referred to as scattering in epithelial cells), migration in the extracellular matrix (ECM), proliferation and acquisition of polarity. This programme is activated under physiological conditions during organ development and regeneration, axon guidance and wound healing (Birchmeier and Gherardi 1998; Comoglio and Boccaccio 2001; Trusolino and Comoglio 2002). The fate of a particular cell activated for invasive growth is dependent on the tissue type and stage in the organism's development (Longati et al. 2001). Although several cytokines and growth factors (e.g. EGF and FGF) can induce components of invasive growth or may contribute to its onset and maintenance, the spatial and chronological orchestration of the various steps involved are optimally accomplished by PRGFs (HGF and MSP), together with their cellular receptors (Met and Ron, respectively). HGF-Met-mediated invasive growth is essential during mammalian development, as mouse knockouts of either HGF or Met result in embryonic lethality due to defects in placenta, liver, muscle and nerves (Birchmeier and Gherardi 1998).

The most dramatic manifestation of physiological invasive growth, especially evident in embryonic development and tissue regeneration, is *branching morphogenesis*, a program of proliferation, migration and differentiation to form a three-dimensional series of tubules (Brinkmann et al. 1995; Montesano et al. 1991). Several different cell types can undergo intrinsic, tissue-specific branching morphogenetic activities in response to HGF. For example, EpH4 mammary epithelial cells in culture, on stimulation with HGF, form long branches with end buds reminiscent of developing mammary ducts and Capan2 pancreatic carcinoma cells develop large, hollow spheroids lined with a tight layer of epithelial cells which resemble pancreatic ducts (Brinkmann et al. 1995). HGF treatment of primary human mammary organoids, in collagen gel cultures, results in a striking display of extensive branching tubules originating specifically from the myoepithelial subpopulation of mammary epithelial cells (not luminal epithelia) (Niranjan et al. 1995). Axon guidance in neurons can be regarded as a specialised form of invasive growth and branching morphogenesis.

The signalling complexes recruited to activated Met in response to HGF are shown in Fig. 1. Activation of signal transduction is mediated by autophosphorylation of specific tyrosine (Tyr) residues within the intracellular domain after receptor dimerisation (Naldini et al. 1991a). Ligand binding results in a rapid rise in cytosolic free calcium (Baffy et al. 1992) and autophosphorylation of Tyr^{1234} and Tyr^{1235}, located within the activation loop of the tyrosine kinase domain, triggering the intrinsic kinase activity of the receptor (Rodrigues and Park 1994). In addition, phosphorylation of Tyr^{1349} and Tyr^{1356} generates a multisubstrate docking site that is conserved among Met family members (Ponzetto et al. 1994). The sequence surrounding Tyr^{1349} and Tyr^{1356} ($Y^{1349}VHVNATY^{1349}VNV$) forms a docking site which binds signal transducers containing src homology 2 (SH2) domains, phosphotyrosine binding (PTB) domains or Met binding domains (MBD) as well as numerous adaptor proteins which not only recruit additional signal transducers indirectly to Met but also additional adaptor proteins through a variety of modular domains. Thus, for example, activation of the Ras-MAP kinase pathway in response to HGF may be the result of both Met-Grb2-SOS and Met-Shc-Grb2-SOS interactions (comprehensively reviewed Furge et al. 2000) (Fig. 1).

Activation of Ras has been shown to play a central role in the entire invasive growth process by inducing cell movement, disassembly of adherens junctions and enzymatic digestion of the ECM, in addition to stimulating proliferation (reviewed in Comoglio and Boccaccio 2001). Activity of Src downstream of Met is essentially proliferative, and coupling to PI3K alone is sufficient to induce HGF-induced motility (Maina et al. 2001). Branching morphogenesis is believed to be a function of prolonged tyrosine phosphorylation of the multisubstrate adaptor/scaffold protein Grb2-associated binding protein 1 (Gab1) on multiple tyrosines, leading to recruitment of PLCγ and the SHP2 phosphatase, together with activation of the STAT pathway (Boccaccio et al. 1998; Gual et al. 2001; Maroun et al. 2000; Schaeper et al. 2000).

Recent investigations have shown that Met kinase activity can be regulated through other receptors by HGF-independent mechanisms. In several cell types, HGF-induced Met signalling depends absolutely on the presence of specific isoforms of the adhesive receptor CD44 (CD44v6). The extracellular domain of CD44 is required and sufficient for Met autophosphorylation, but the cytoplasmic domain is required for transmitting the signal from activated Met to MEK (MAP kinase kinase) and ERK (MAP kinase) (Orian-Rousseau et al. 2002). In a variety of carcinoma cells, HGF-dependent invasion requires a physical association between Met and the $\alpha_6\beta_4$-integrin at the plasma membrane. Activation of Met results not only in tyrosine phosphorylation of its own intracellular domain but also tyrosine phosphorylation of the integrin β_4 cytoplasmic domain, thus creating an additional docking platform for intracellular transducers which cooperate with Met to potentiate downstream targets in order to achieve full execution of Met-dependent responses (Trusolino et al. 2001). Similarly, in certain epithelial cell lines, invasive growth mediated by plexin B1 is dependent upon a physical association of its receptor (semaphorin 4D) with Met. In this case, binding of ligand (plexin) to semaphorin 4D stimulates not only semaphorin 4D autophosphorylation but phosphorylation of Met as well (Giordano et al. 2002). Pre-existing, ligand-independent heterodimers between Met and its homologue Ron have also been detected on the cell surface (Follenzi et al. 2000) and may be able to transphosphorylate one another. Interactions between Met and additional RTK family members [e.g. EGF receptor (EGFR)] have also been demonstrated in transformed cells (Jo et al. 2000).

1.3
Aberrant Invasive Growth: The Malignant Phenotype

Aberrant HGF-Met signalling is widely implicated in the generation and spread of tumours and metastases. The most convincing evidence of the involvement of Met in human cancer has been obtained from analysis of patients affected by hereditary papillary renal carcinoma (HPRC). A number of distinct germ line mutations in the Met tyrosine kinase domain have been identified in specific cases of HPRC, all of which result in hyperactivation of Met (Olivero et al. 1999; Schmidt et al. 1997). Met and/or HGF expression or overexpression has been documented in a wide variety of other tumour types, including hepatocellular carcinomas, head and neck squamous cell carcinomas and gastric carcinoma (Jeffers et al. 1997a; reviewed in Danilkovitch-Miagkova and Zbar 2002; Jeffers et al. 1996).

The process of metastasis, when neoplastic cells leave their primary site of accretion, cross tissue boundaries and enter the vasculature to colonise distant sites, can be regarded as the aberrant counterpart of invasive growth (Jeffers et al. 1996; Trusolino and Comoglio 2002). Constitutive upregulation of Met activity correlates with the metastatic ability of tumour cells (Haddad et al. 2001). Under malignant neoplastic conditions, the growth-promoting (mitogenic) activity of Met causes cellular transformation, whereas its ability to enhance motility (morphogenic and motogenic) and survival (anti-apoptotic) accounts for cellular invasion and metastasis. The signalling pathways involved are likely to be the same during tumour development and progression as under physiological conditions—they will simply be deregulated. The concept that Met drives cells to invade and to form metastases has been validated in several model systems, especially mouse models using both transfected cells (Giordano et al. 1997; Meiners et al. 1998; Rong et al. 1993) and transgenic animals (Jeffers et al. 1998; Liang et al. 1996; Otsuka et al. 1998) (reviewed in Jeffers et al. 1996).

The various mechanisms through which aberrant Met activation can contribute to tumourigenesis are highlighted in Fig. 2. As well as the well-defined routes to enhancement of Met signalling through gene translocations, activating mutations and amplification, defects in negative regulators of Met in certain cancer cells are believed to contribute to oncogenesis (Fig. 2B). Recent studies have revealed that negative signalling by RTKs involves the coordinated action of ubiquitin ligases (e.g. Cbl), adaptor proteins (e.g. Grb2 and CIN85), inhibitory molecules (e.g. Sprouty), cytoplasmic kinases and phosphoinositol metabolites (Dikic and Giordano 2003; Peschard and Park 2003). In metastatic B16 melanoma cells, cytosolic phosphatases that normally mediate Met dephosphorylation are downregulated, leading to constitutive Met activation (Rusciano et al. 1996).

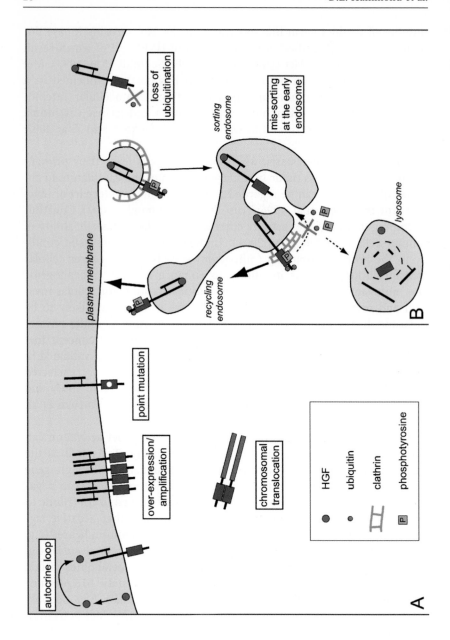

2
Receptor Trafficking

Stimulation of RTKs not only elicits receptor autophosphorylation and phosphorylation of intracellular substrates but also triggers internalisation of receptor-ligand complexes in clathrin-coated vesicles by receptor-mediated endocytosis. Internalised receptors are then either recycled back to the plasma membrane or targeted for degradation in lysosomes. This *downregulation* serves to reduce the number of activated receptors, thereby attenuating receptor signalling. The EGFR provides the paradigm for membrane trafficking of RTKs, in part owing to elegant electron microscopic studies (Felder et al. 1990; Futter et al. 2001; Longva et al. 2002; Sachse et al. 2002).These have revealed that lysosomally directed receptor is sequestered from the cytosol by inclusion in small vesicles which pinch off the limiting membrane into the lumen of sorting endosomes to generate multivesicular bodies (MVBs), which then deliver material to lysosomes for degradation. Recent advances have highlighted multiple roles for ubiquitin on the endocytic pathway and the involvement of many proteins containing domains that specify ubiquitin interaction (e.g. UIM, CUE) (Schnell and Hicke 2003). Of particular note, the UIM-containing hepatocyte growth factor regulated tyrosine kinase substrate (Hrs) is proposed to act as an adaptor at the endosomal membrane, linking ubiquitinated receptors to the endosomal sorting complex required for transport (ESCRT) machinery that promotes this luminal budding (Clague 2002; Raiborg et al. 2002; Sachse et al. 2002).

◀───

Fig. 2A, B. Mechanisms through which Met activation can be deregulated in tumour cells. **A** Uncontrolled Met signalling can be caused by improper autocrine or paracrine stimulation, receptor and/or ligand overexpression or amplification, activating mutations and chromosomal translocations (e.g. *tpr-met*). **B** It is now apparent that loss of negative regulators of Met may be as important as a gain of positive activating mutation(s) in contributing to oncogenesis. For example, a loss of Cbl-dependent ubiquitination of Met after stimulation, and hence prevention of degradation/downregulation is another mechanism whereby the receptor can be deregulated in cancer (Peschard and Park 2003). In addition, we propose that aberrant Met signalling may arise as a consequence of defective trafficking of activated Met towards degradation due to mis-sorting at the early endosome (Hammond et al. 2003; see text for details)

2.1
Met Degradation Is Sensitive to Proteasome Inhibition

In common with many RTKs, Met receptor is ubiquitinated after stimulation. The presence of a polyubiquitin chain comprised of at least four monomers generally targets proteins to be degraded by the 26S proteasome (Deveraux et al. 1994). HGF-dependent Met degradation is exquisitely sensitive to proteasome inhibitors such as lactacystin or MG132, a property which is not shared with other well-studied RTKs which are nevertheless ubiquitinated (e.g. EGFR). This observation led Jeffers et al. to conclude that Met receptor is directly degraded by the proteasome (Jeffers et al. 1997b). However, further studies from our laboratory showed that in HeLa cells, indirect inhibition of lysosomal acid-dependent proteases with proton pump inhibitors (e.g. concanamycin) also provided a significant block to HGF-dependent Met degradation (Hammond et al. 2001). Thus the proteasome inhibitor-sensitive pathway of Met degradation must overlap with the endosomal pathway. Contrary results have been reported by Kermorgant et al. who confirmed that Met degradation is proteasome dependent but failed to detect any inhibition by concanamycin (Kermorgant et al. 2003).

Hammond et al. further showed that expression of a dominant-negative form of dynamin (K44A) in HeLa cells, which inhibits the major endocytic pathways at the plasma membrane, significantly slows Met degradation without providing a complete block. Simple kinetic considerations suggested that in normal HeLa cells, after acute HGF stimulation, two-thirds of Met receptors will be degraded by a proteasome-dependent endosomal pathway. The remaining one-third is degraded by a poorly defined, proteasome-dependent pathway, which is insensitive to proton pump inhibitors (Hammond et al. 2001).

2.2
Proteasome Inhibitors Perturb HGF-Dependent Met Trafficking

Using fluorescence microscopy of HeLa cells fixed after acute stimulation with HGF, Hammond et al. observed a time-dependent redistribution of the Met receptor consistent with entry into the endosomal pathway and delivery to perinuclear late endosomal compartments (Hammond et al. 2001). Prior treatment of cells with proteasome inhibitors blocked this HGF-dependent redistribution from the plasma membrane without affecting other receptor trafficking itineraries (transferrin receptor, EGFR). Biochemical measurement of Met internalisation rates showed no change due to proteasomal inhibition; rather, lactacystin treatment promotes fast recycling of Met to the plasma membrane (Hammond et al. 2003). Thus possibly the major means by which proteasome inhibitors inhibit HGF-dependent Met degradation is by rerouting internalised receptors from the MVB-lysosome pathway to the plasma membrane recycling pathway (Fig. 2B).

Although ligand-dependent degradation of many RTK receptors such as EGFR and PDGFR is largely insensitive to proteasome inhibitors (Bonifacino and Weissman 1998), other non-RTK receptors such as IL-2 and growth hormone receptor (GHR) show similar sensitivities (Rocca et al. 2001; van Kerkhof et al. 2000). Even in the case of EGFR, Longva et al. showed that lactacystin inhibits incorporation of EGFR into luminal vesicles of MVBs (Longva et al. 2002). Nevertheless, it appears that EGFR gets sorted to the limiting membrane of late endosomes, where it can be partially degraded. Thus in EGFR there may be a hierarchy of sorting signals to late endosomes that is absent in the Met receptor.

2.3
Cellular Factors Which Determine Met Trafficking

It is only in the last 3 years that Met receptor endocytosis has been subject to study; therefore, many of our assumptions are still based on data from more extensively studied receptors. Met enters cells through a dynamin-dependent process which is most likely to be a clathrin-coated vesicle pathway (Hammond et al. 2001). The E3 ubiquitin ligase, Cbl, is recruited to activated receptor and serves as an adaptor protein mediating recruitment of two other factors which appear necessary for both Met and EGFR internalisation, CIN85 (Cbl-interacting protein of 85 kDa) and endophilin (Petrelli et al. 2002; Soubeyran et al. 2002). Petrelli et al. could impair Met receptor internalisation by expression of dominant interfering forms of each component of this complex. Endophilin possesses fatty acid transferase activity, which has been proposed to promote receptor endocytosis by inducing negative curvature in membranes at the neck of the budding vesicle, thereby reducing an energy barrier to fission (Farsad et al. 2001; Schmidt et al. 1999). However, intriguing recent reports also link this complex to actin organisation, which has been shown to be an essential factor in clathrin-mediated endocytosis. Endophilin interacts with neural Wiskott-Aldrich syndrome protein (N-WASP) after EGF stimulation and enhances N-WASP-induced actin-related protein 2/3 (Arp 2/3) activity in vitro (Otsuki et al. 2003). Cortactin, which regulates the formation of dynamic actin networks via the Arp2/3 complex, has been identified as a binding partner for the CIN85-related protein CD2AP (Lynch et al. 2003).

Separate from its role as an adaptor protein, Cbl is also directly responsible for Met receptor ubiquitination. This may occur either at the plasma membrane or at the sorting endosome. The reaction requires a functional SH2 domain and a RING domain within Cbl (Peschard et al. 2001). Cbl is recruited to activated phospho-Tyr[1356] of Met via Grb2, but then subsequent binding of its TKB domain to the juxtamembrane autophosphorylated Tyr[1003] is proposed to elicit a conformational change within Cbl necessary for activation. A Y1003F mutation inhibits ligand-dependent ubiquitination of Met and leads to cell transformation (Peschard et al. 2001).

Ubiquitination of RTKs results in up-shifted smearing of bands on electrophoresis gels and was previously believed to represent polyubiquitination of receptors such as EGFR (Galcheva-Gargova et al. 1995) and PDGFR (Mori et al. 1992). However, it was shown recently that the downregulation of EGFR and PDGFR actually involves the addition of single ubiquitin monomers to multiple lysine residues within the C-termini of the receptors (termed multiple monoubiquitination) (Haglund et al. 2003; Mosesson et al. 2003). Preliminary data from our laboratory also suggest that the polyubiquitination of Met actually represents a similar multiple monoubiquitination of the receptor. This has led to the proposal that there may be a conserved mechanism to limit the E3 ligase activity of Cbl to monoubiquitination. Receptor monoubiquitination is sufficient for engagement with the sorting machinery necessary for delivery to MVBs, a process which is most likely mediated through interaction with the UIM domain of Hrs.

3
Relationship Between Endocytic Trafficking and Met Receptor Signalling

EGFR typically recycles through the sorting or early endosome three to five times before it is selected for degradation in a stochastic manner by routing to late endosomal compartments. At steady state 70%–80% of the EGF-occupied EGFR is endosomal (Sorkin 1998). Several lines of evidence support the view that the receptor can maintain its signalling status during a substantial part of this cycle (reviewed in Clague and Urbe 2001; Sorkin and von Zastrow 2002).

Subcellular localisation can determine the exposure of activated receptors to different effector molecules and determine the relative strengths of particular signalling outputs. For EGFR, this was most elegantly shown by induction of mutant dynamin, under the control of a tetracycline switch, to block receptor internalisation. Vieria et al. clearly demonstrated changes to the EGF signalling profile when EGFR endocytosis was blocked by this method (Vieria et al. 1996). Since then, this approach has been used with a variety of RTKs and G protein receptors (Sorkin and von Zastrow 2002).

Acute stimulation of Met with HGF results in receptor autophosphorylation on tyrosine residues which normally peaks within 10 min, and subsequently attenuates—that is, Met becomes dephosphorylated. In some cell types, Met dephosphorylation can be kinetically dissociated from ligand-induced Met degradation (Hammond et al. 2003). Petrelli et al. used interfering forms of endophilin A3 to block endocytosis in HEK 293T cells and observed extended Met phosphorylation as well as sustained Gab1 phosphorylation. Expression of dominant interfering forms of endophilin A3 or CIN85 also increased HGF-dependent chemotaxis of HEK 293T cells (Petrelli et al. 2002). Similar results were obtained in HeLa cells after expression of dominant-negative dynamin (Hammond et al. 2003). Furthermore, the Y1003F mutant form of Met that is deficient in Cbl ubiquitin ligase activation shows enhanced phosphorylation (Peschard and Park 2003).

We have taken advantage of our observation that proteasome inhibitors perturb Met endocytic trafficking after internalisation to ask for the first time whether endosomal sorting also influences signalling output of an activated receptor. In cells treated with the proteasome inhibitor lactacystin we observe a failure of both Met dephosphorylation and Met degradation (Hammond et al. 2003). We cannot completely rule out that lactacystin may be directly affecting the dephosphorylation of Met by an as yet unknown mechanism, but it seems most likely that the effect of lactacystin on ligand-induced Met phosphorylation is due to its influence on Met dynamics. Lactacystin treatment recapitulates the sustained phosphorylation of receptor observed after expression of dominant-negative (K44A) dynamin or endophilin. It therefore appears that internalisation is not a prerequisite for maximum phosphorylation of Met but both internalisation and correct partitioning within, or retention at, the sorting endosome are required for Met dephosphorylation. Similar perturbation of GHR dynamics by lactacystin has been shown to result in stabilisation of GHR and downstream JAK2 tyrosine phosphorylation (Alves dos Santos et al. 2001).

Our data is consistent with Met having restricted access to a specific protein tyrosine phosphatase (PTP) under conditions of proteasome inhibition. This phosphatase must be located downstream of early endosomal sorting but must not be able to diffuse freely throughout the cell, because inhibiting the correct sorting of Met to degradative late endosomal/lysosomal compartments of the endocytic pathway with proteasome inhibitors prevents Met dephosphorylation. Interestingly, ligand-induced trafficking of activated EGFR and PDGFβR and their dephosphorylation by the ER-resident phosphatase PTP1B have recently been visualised (Haj et al. 2002). Correct endosomal sorting of Met to access the same (or similar) ER PTP may be required for its dephosphorylation. Aside from the promiscuous transmembrane PTP leukocyte antigen-related protein (Kulas et al. 1996) and the soluble phosphatase PTP-S (Villa-Moruzzi et al. 1998), very few specific modulators of HGF-induced Met activation have been identified except for the PTP DEP-1 (CD148/PTP-η) (Palka et al. 2003). DEP-1 was recently shown to form a stable complex with CSF-Met, a chimeric receptor consisting of the extracellular domain of the colony-stimulating factor 1 (CSF) receptor and the Met intracellular domain. Furthermore, DEP-1 preferentially dephosphorylates Tyr^{1349} of Met as well as an additional C-terminal Tyr^{1365} implicated in branching morphogenesis, thus potentially providing an additional mechanism through which signal specificity through Met may be conferred (Palka et al. 2003).

The Ras-MAPK kinase pathway controls both HGF-dependent proliferation and motility (Hartmann et al. 1994; Ponzetto et al. 1994; Potempa and Ridley 1998; Ridley et al. 1995; Tanimura et al. 1998). Analysis in HeLa cells of the time-dependent phosphorylation profile of ERK and its upstream partner MEK after acute administration of HGF demonstrate that both are transiently phosphorylated and that both the initial response and subsequent attenuation are insensitive to disrupted Met trafficking through either perturbation of early endosomal sorting (lactacystin treatment) or inhibition of internalisation (overexpression of K44A dynamin) (Hammond et al. 2003). Thus, rather counterintuitively, attenuation of Ras-MAPK signalling can proceed in the face of sustained activation of the Met receptor itself. This implies that the PTP(s) responsible for the dephosphorylation of ERK and MEK must be distinct from that required for dephosphorylation of Met itself. They must also be able to both gain access to their substrates and function in a sustained manner, to suppress the ERK and MEK response to continued Met activation.

The prominent HGF receptor tyrosine kinase substrate, Hrs, is an early endosome localised protein which requires coincident localisation with receptors at the sorting endosome for efficient phosphorylation to occur (Hammond et al. 2003; Komada et al. 1997; Urbé et al. 2000). It is highly concentrated in regions of the vacuolar sorting endosome which are covered with a *bilayered* clathrin coat where lysosomally directed receptors (GHR and EGFR) are also concentrated, perhaps through interaction with the UIM domain of Hrs (Sachse et al. 2002). We have shown that dynamin-dependent endocytosis of receptor must occur for efficient phosphorylation of Hrs after EGF (Urbé et al. 2000) and HGF stimulation (Hammond et al. 2003). A striking difference exists, however, between the effects of proteasome inhibition on phosphorylation of Hrs in response to either HGF or EGF. Lactacytsin treatment dramatically inhibits HGF-dependent phosphorylation of Hrs but, curiously, not EGF-dependent phosphorylation of Hrs. Indeed, EGF-induced Hrs phosphorylation actually increases at extended time points after addition of ligand (20 min). Lactacystin has previously been shown to reduce GHR concentration in the clathrin-coated regions of endosomes (Sachse et al. 2002). We propose that lactacystin is similarly inhibiting Met concentration (but not EGFR) in this coated region, thereby denying access to its substrate Hrs (Hammond et al. 2003). Future work will test this proposal with electron microscopy. We also speculate that this differential effect on Hrs phosphorylation may be directly related to the differential effect of lactacystin on Met versus EGFR degradation. Failure to be retained within the coated regions may release Met receptors to the recycling pathway. RNAi- mediated knockdown of Hrs in HeLa cells modestly retarded Met degradation but had a more pronounced effect on Met dephosphorylation. This observation reinforces the findings obtained with lactacystin treatment that correct partitioning within sorting endosomes, probably to bilayered clathrin-coated areas, facilitates both Met dephosphorylation and degradation (Hammond et al. 2003).

4
The Endocytic Pathway as a Tumour Suppressor System

Endocytosis of activated RTKs represents the major pathway for down-regulation and can also influence signalling outputs. The endocytic pathway can therefore be proposed to be a tumour suppressor pathway, inactivation of which may promote cellular transformation (Clague and Urbe 2001; Di Fiore and Gill 1999).

This idea is supported by a number of observations regarding the Cbl family of E3 ubiquitin ligases. Cbl is a proto-oncogene which was first identified in a retrovirus which induced haematopoietic tumours in mice. This oncogenic form of Cbl (termed v-Cbl) is a truncated protein which lacks ubiquitin ligase activity and is able to compete with wild-type Cbl for binding sites on activated RTKs and consequently inhibits receptor downregulation (reviewed in Thien et al. 2001). It has been demonstrated that the mutation of a tyrosine residue within the jux-tamembrane domain of Met (Y1003F) produces a receptor which can no longer bind Cbl and which therefore is no longer ubiquitinated. This mutant receptor has been shown to have a prolonged half-life and to possess transforming ability (Peschard et al. 2001). Similar mutations have also been identified in other receptors (i.e. c-Kit, EGFR and CSF-1R) which prevent Cbl binding and also have transforming ability (re-viewed in Peschard and Park 2003).

A second endocytic protein which has been implicated in tumourige-nesis is the clathrin assembly lymphoid myeloid leukaemia (CALM) pro-tein. CALM is a non-neuronal homologue of the synaptic protein AP180 which is known to be involved in clathrin coat assembly and endocytic vesicle formation at the plasma membrane of nerve termini. CALM itself has been implicated in clathrin-mediated endocytosis after observations that it is located in clathrin-coated areas of the plasma membrane and that overexpression leads to inhibition of transferrin receptor and EGFR endocytosis (Tebar et al. 1999). CALM was initially identified as part of a fusion protein which results from a chromosomal abnormality found in patients with acute lymphoblastic or acute myeloid leukaemias (Dreyling et al. 1996). This fusion protein is composed of almost the en-tire CALM protein fused to the a small portion of a putative transcrip-tion factor called AF10. This CALM-AF10 fusion protein has since been detected in a number of leukaemias, and a second CALM fusion protein (MLL-CALM) has also been detected in a case of acute myeloid leukae-mia (Wechsler et al. 2003). Leukaemias associated with CALM fusion proteins are aggressive and have a poor prognosis (Bohlander et al. 2000; Wechsler et al. 2003). It has been proposed that the formation of these CALM fusion proteins may inhibit the normal function of CALM and may therefore perturb the clathrin-mediated endocytosis of growth factor receptors, resulting in persistent growth factor signalling (Wechsler et al. 2003).

Tumour susceptibility gene 101 (TSG101), a component of ESCRT 1 implicated in promotion of MVB formation (Katzmann et al. 2001), was originally discovered by its ability to neoplastically transform mouse

3T3 cells when deficient or overexpressed (Li and Cohen 1996). Mouse fibroblast SL6 cells, which are deficient in TSG101, were found to have defects in their delivery of EGFR to late endosomal compartments (Babst et al. 2000). siRNA-mediated knock-down of TSG101 in human cells also leads to accumulation of EGFR due to failure of the degradation pathway (Bishop et al. 2002).

Transforming mutations of EGFR that are defective in endocytic trafficking were characterised previously (Wells et al. 1990), although they have not formally been shown to be oncogenic in 'standard' model systems used to assess malignancy, nor have they been isolated from primary tumours. The recent discovery of a novel germ line Met mutation (P991S) in a primary gastric cancer is interesting (Lee et al. 2000). All previous naturally occurring Met mutations which have transforming activity have been found within the tyrosine kinase domain of the receptor and either are constitutively active or possess a reduced threshold for activation (Chiara et al. 2003). In contrast, P991S Met contains a mutation within the juxtamembrane domain of the receptor and does not exhibit enhanced tyrosine kinase activity. However, once stimulated with HGF, the receptor shows increased and prolonged phosphorylation compared to wild-type receptors (Lee et al. 2000). Future studies will determine whether this mutation leads to defective endocytic trafficking of the receptor and a firm example of the link between the endocytic pathway and cancer.

References

Alves dos Santos CM, van Kerkhof P, and Strous GJ (2001) The signal transduction of the growth hormone receptor is regulated by the ubiquitin/proteasome system and continues after endocytosis. J Biol Chem 276, 10839–10846

Babst M, Odorizzi G, Estepa EJ, and Emr SD (2000) Mammalian tumour susceptibility gene 101 (TSG101) and the yeast homologue, Vps23p, both function in late endosomal trafficking. Traffic 1, 248–258

Baffy G, Yang L, Michalopoulos GK, and Williamson JR (1992) Hepatocyte growth factor induces calcium mobilization and inositol phosphate production in rat hepatocytes. J Cell Physiol 153, 332–339

Birchmeier C, and Gherardi E (1998) Developmental roles of HGF/SF and its receptor, the c-Met tyrosine kinase. Trends Cell Biol 8, 404–410

Bishop N, Horman A, and Woodman P (2002) Mammalian class E vps proteins recognize ubiquitin and act in the removal of endosomal protein-ubiquitin conjugates. J Cell Biol 157, 91–101

Boccaccio C, Ando M, Tamagnone L, Bardelli A, Michieli P, Battistini C, and Comoglio PM (1998) Induction of epithelial tubules by growth factor HGF depends on the STAT pathway. Nature 391, 285–288

Bohlander SK, Muschinsky V, Schrader K, Siebert R, Schlegelberger B, Harder L, Schemmel V, Fonatsch C, Ludwig WD, Hiddemann W, and Dreyling MH (2000) Molecular analysis of the CALM/AF10 fusion: identical rearrangements in acute myeloid leukemia, acute lymphoblastic leukemia and malignant lymphoma patients. Leukemia 14, 93–99

Bonifacino JS, and Weissman A (1998) Ubiquitin and the control of protein fate in the secretory and endocytic pathways. Annu Rev Cell Dev Biol 14, 19–57

Bottaro DP, Rubin JS, Faletto DL, Chan AM, Kmiecik TE, Vande Woude GF, and Aaronson SA (1991) Identification of the hepatocyte growth factor receptor as the c-met oncogene product. Science 251, 802–804

Brinkmann V, Foroutan H, Sachs M, Weidner KM, and Birchmeier W (1995) Hepatocyte growth factor/scatter factor induces a variety of tissue-specific morphogenic programs in epithelial cells. J Cell Biol 131, 1573–1586

Chiara F, Michieli P, Pugliese L, and Comoglio PM (2003) Mutations in the met oncogene unveil a "dual switch" mechanism controlling tyrosine kinase activity. J Biol Chem 278, 29352–29358

Clague MJ (2002) Membrane transport: a coat for ubiquitin. Curr Biol 12, R529–R531

Clague MJ, and Urbe S (2001) The interface of receptor trafficking and signalling. J Cell Sci 114, 3075–3081

Comoglio PM, and Boccaccio C (2001) Scatter factors and invasive growth. Semin Cancer Biol 11, 153–165

Comoglio PM, and Trusolino L (2002) Invasive growth: from development to metastasis. J Clin Invest 109, 857–862

Cooper CS, Park M, Blair DG, Tainsky MA, Huebner K, Croce CM, and Vande Woude GF (1984) Molecular cloning of a new transforming gene from a chemically transformed cell line. Nature 311, 29–33

Danilkovitch-Miagkova A, and Zbar B (2002) Dysregulation of Met receptor tyrosine kinase activity in invasive tumors. J Clin Invest 109, 863–867

Dean M, Park M, Le Beau MM, Robins TS, Diaz MO, Rowley JD, Blair DG, and Vande Woude GF (1985) The human met oncogene is related to the tyrosine kinase oncogenes. Nature 318, 385–388

Deveraux Q, Ustrell V, Pickart C, and Rechsteiner M (1994) A 26 S protease subunit that binds ubiquitin conjugates. J Biol Chem 269, 7059–7061

Di Fiore PP, and Gill GN (1999) Endocytosis and mitogenic signalling. Curr Opin Cell Biol 11, 483–488

Dikic I, and Giordano S (2003) Negative receptor signalling. Curr Opin Cell Biol 15, 128–135

Dreyling MH, Martinez-Climent JA, Zheng M, Mao J, Rowley JD, and Bohlander SK (1996) The t(10;11)(p13;q14) in the U937 cell line results in the fusion of the AF10 gene and CALM, encoding a new member of the AP-3 clathrin assembly protein family. Proc Natl Acad Sci U S A 93, 4804–4809

Farsad K, Ringstad N, Takei K, Floyd SR, Rose K, and De Camilli P (2001) Generation of high curvature membranes mediated by direct endophilin bilayer interactions. J Cell Biol 155, 193–200

Felder S, Miller K, Moehren G, Ullrich A, Schlessinger J, and Hopkins CR (1990) Kinase activity controls the sorting of the epidermal growth factor receptor within the multivesicular body. Cell 61, 623–634

Follenzi A, Bakovic S, Gual P, Stella MC, Longati P, and Comoglio PM (2000) Crosstalk between the proto-oncogenes Met and Ron. Oncogene 19, 3041–3049

Furge KA, Zhang Y-W, and Vande Woude GF (2000) Met receptor tyrosine kinase: enhanced signaling through adaptor proteins. Oncogene 19, 5582–5589

Futter CE, Collinson LM, Backer JM, and Hopkins CR (2001) Human VPS34 is required for internal vesicle formation within multivesicular endosomes. J Cell Biol 155, 1251–1264

Galcheva-Gargova Z, Theroux SJ, and Davis RJ (1995) The epidermal growth factor receptor is covalently linked to ubiquitin. Oncogene 11, 2649–2655

Gaudino G, Follenzi A, Naldini L, Collesi C, Santoro M, Gallo KA, Godowski PJ, and Comoglio PM (1994) RON is a heterodimeric tyrosine kinase receptor activated by the HGF homologue MSP. EMBO J 13, 3524–3532

Giordano S, Bardelli A, Zhen Z, Menard S, Ponzetto C, and Comoglio PM (1997) A point mutation in the MET oncogene abrogates metastasis without affecting transformation. Proc Natl Acad Sci U S A 94, 13868–13872

Giordano S, Corso S, Conrotto P, Artigiani S, Gilestro G, Barberis D, Tamagnone L, and Comoglio PM (2002) The semaphorin 4D receptor controls invasive growth by coupling with Met. Nat Cell Biol 4, 720–724

Giordano S, Di Renzo MF, Narsimhan RP, Cooper CS, Rosa C, and Comoglio PM (1989) Oncogene 4, 1383–1388

Gual P, Giordano S, Anguissola S, Parker PJ, and Comoglio PM (2001) Gab1 phosphorylation: a novel mechanism for negative regulation of HGF receptor signaling. Oncogene 20, 156–166

Haddad R, Lipson KE, and Webb CP (2001) Hepatocyte growth factor expression in human cancer and therapy with specific inhibitors. Anticancer Res 21, 4243–4252

Haglund K, Sigismund S, Polo S, Szymkiewicz I, Di Fiore PP, and Dikic I (2003) Multiple monoubiquitination of RTKs is sufficient for their endocytosis and degradation. Nat Cell Biol 5, 461–466

Haj FG, Verveer PJ, Squire A, Neel BG, and Bastiaens PI (2002) Imaging sites of receptor dephosphorylation by PTP1B on the surface of the endoplasmic reticulum. Science 295, 1708–1711

Hammond DE, Carter S, McCullough J, Urbe S, Vande Woude G, and Clague MJ (2003) Endosomal dynamics of met determine signaling output. Mol Biol Cell 14, 1346–1354

Hammond DE, Urbe S, Vande Woude GF, and Clague MJ (2001) Down-regulation of MET, the receptor for hepatocyte growth factor. Oncogene 20, 2761–2770

Hartmann G, Weidner KM, Schwarz H, and Birchmeier W (1994) The motility signal of scatter factor/hepatocyte growth factor mediated through the receptor tyrosine kinase met requires intracellular action of Ras. J Biol Chem 269, 21936–21939

Jeffers M, Fiscella M, Webb CP, Anver M, Koochekpour S, and Vande Woude GF (1998) The mutationally activated Met receptor mediates motility and metastasis. Proc Natl Acad Sci U S A 95, 14417–14422

Jeffers M, Rong S, and Vande Woude GF (1996) Hepatocyte growth factor/scatter factor-Met signaling in tumorigenicity and invasion/metastasis. J Mol Med 74, 505–513

Jeffers M, Schmidt L, Nakaigawa N, Webb CP, Weirich G, Kishida T, Zbar B, and Vande Woude GF (1997a) Activating mutations for the Met tyrosine kinase receptor in human cancer. Proc Natl Acad Sci USA 94, 11445–11450

Jeffers M, Taylor GA, Weidner KM, Omura S, and Vande Woude GF (1997b) Degradation of the Met tyrosine kinase receptor by the ubiquitin-proteasome pathway. Mol Cell Biol 17, 799–808

Jo M, Stolz DB, Esplen JE, Dorko K, Michalopoulos GK, and Strom SC (2000) Crosstalk between epidermal growth factor receptor and c-Met signal pathways in transformed cells. J Biol Chem 275, 8806–8811

Katzmann DJ, Babst M, and Emr SD (2001) Ubiquitin-dependent sorting into the multivesicular body pathway requires the function of a conserved endosomal protein sorting complex, ESCRT-1. Cell 106, 145–155

Kermorgant S, Zicha D, and Parker PJ (2003) Protein kinase C controls microtubule-based traffic but not proteasomal degradation of c-Met. J Biol Chem 278, 28921–28929

Komada M, Masaki R, Yamamoto A, and Kitamura N (1997) Hrs, a tyrosine kinase substrate with a conserved double zinc finger domain, is localized to the cytoplasmic surface of early endosomes. J Biol Chem 272, 20538–20544

Kulas DT, Goldstein BJ, and Mooney RA (1996) The transmembrane protein-tyrosine phosphatase LAR modulates signaling by multiple receptor tyrosine kinases. J Biol Chem 271, 748–754

Lee J-H, Han S-U, Cho H, Jennings B, Gerrard B, Dean M, Schmidt L, Zbar B, and Vande Woude GF (2000) A novel germ line juxtamembrane Met mutation in human gastric cancer. Oncogene 19, 4947–4953

Li L, and Cohen SN (1996) Tsg101: a novel tumor susceptibility gene isolated by controlled homozygous functional knockout of allelic loci in mammalian cells. Cell 85, 319–329

Liang TJ, Reid AE, Xavier R, Cardiff RD, and Wang TC (1996) Transgenic expression of tpr-met oncogene leads to development of mammary hyperplasia and tumors. J Clin Invest 97, 2872–2877

Longati P, Comoglio PM, and Bardelli A (2001) Receptor tyrosine kinases as therapeutic targets: the model of the MET oncogene. Curr Drug Targets 2, 41–55

Longva KE, Blystad FD, Stang E, Larsen A, M, Johannessen LE, and Madshus IH (2002) Ubiquitination and proteasomal activity is required for transport of the EGF receptor to inner membranes of multivesicular bodies. J Cell Biol 156, 843–854

Lynch DK, Winata SC, Lyons RJ, Hughes WE, Lehrbach GM, Wasinger V, Corthals G, Cordwell S, and Daly RJ (2003) A Cortactin-CD2-associated protein (CD2AP) complex provides a novel link between epidermal growth factor receptor endocytosis and the actin cytoskeleton. J Biol Chem 278, 21805–21813

Maina F, Pante G, Helmbacher F, Andres R, Porthin A, Davies AM, Ponzetto C, and Klein R (2001) Coupling Met to specific pathways results in distinct developmental outcomes. Mol Cell 7, 1293–1306

Maroun CR, Naujokas MA, Holgado-Madruga M, Wong AJ, and Park M (2000) The tyrosine phosphatase SHP-2 is required for sustained activation of extracellular signal-regulated kinase and epithelial morphogenesis downstream from the met receptor tyrosine kinase. Mol Cell Biol 20, 8513–8525

Matsumoto K, Kataoka H, Date K, and Nakamura T (1998) Cooperative interaction between alpha- and beta-chains of hepatocyte growth factor on c-Met receptor confers ligand-induced receptor tyrosine phosphorylation and multiple biological responses. J Biol Chem 273, 22913–22920

Meiners S, Brinkmann V, Naundorf H, and Birchmeier W (1998) Role of morphogenetic factors in metastasis of mammary carcinoma cells. Oncogene 16, 9–20

Montesano R, Schaller G, and Orci L (1991) Induction of epithelial tubular morphogenesis in vitro by fibroblast-derived soluble factors. Cell 66, 697–711

Mori S, Heldin C-H, and Claesson-Welsh L (1992) Ligand-induced plyubiquitination of the platelet derived growth factor b-receptor. J Biol Chem 267, 6429–6434

Mosesson Y, Shtiegman K, Katz M, Zwang Y, Vereb G, Szollosi J, and Yarden Y (2003) Endocytosis of receptor tyrosine kinases is driven by monoubiquitylation, not polyubiquitylation. J Biol Chem 278, 21323–21326

Naka D, Ishii T, Yoshiyama Y, Miyazawa K, Hara H, Hishida T, and Kidamura N (1992) Activation of hepatocyte growth factor by proteolytic conversion of a single chain form to a heterodimer. J Biol Chem 267, 20114–20119

Nakamura T, Nawa K, and Ichihara A (1984) Partial purification and characterization of hepatocyte growth factor from serum of hepatectomized rats. Biochem Biophys Res Commun 122, 1450–1459

Naldini L, Vigna E, Ferracini R, Longati P, Gandino L, Prat M, and Comoglio PM (1991a) The tyrosine kinase encoded by the MET proto-oncogene is activated by autophosphorylation. Mol Cell Biol 11, 1793–1803

Naldini L, Weidner KM, Vigna G, Gaudino G, Bardelli A, Ponzetto C, Narsimhan RP, Hartmann G, Zarnegar R, Michalopoulos GK, et al. (1991b) Scatter factor and hepatocyte growth factor are indistinguishable ligands for the MET receptor. EMBO J 10, 2867–2878

Niranjan B, Buluwela L, Yant J, Perusinghe N, Atherton A, Phippard D, Dale T, Gusterson B, and Kamalati T (1995) HGF/SF: a potent cytokine for mammary growth, morphogenesis and development. Development 121, 2897–2908

Olivero M, Valente G, Bardelli A, Longati P, Ferrero N, Cracco C, Terrone C, Rocca-Rossetti S, Comoglio PM, and Di Renzo MF (1999) Novel mutation in the ATP-binding site of the MET oncogene tyrosine kinase in a HPRCC family. Int J Cancer 82, 640–643

Orian-Rousseau V, Chen L, Sleeman JP, Herrlich P, and Ponta H (2002) CD44 is required for two consecutive steps in HGF/c-Met signaling. Genes Dev 16, 3074–3086

Otsuka T, Takayama H, Sharp R, Celli G, LaRochelle WJ, Bottaro DP, Ellmore N, Vieira W, Owens JW, Anver M, and Merlino G (1998) c-Met autocrine activation induces development of malignant melanoma and acquisition of the metastatic phenotype. Cancer Res 58, 5157–5167

Otsuki M, Itoh T, and Takenawa T (2003) Neural Wiskott-Aldrich syndrome protein is recruited to rafts and associates with endophilin A in response to epidermal growth factor. J Biol Chem 278, 6461–6469

Palka HL, Park M, and Tonks NK (2003) Hepatocyte growth factor receptor tyrosine kinase met is a substrate of the receptor protein-tyrosine phosphatase DEP-1. J Biol Chem 278, 5728–5735

Park M, Dean M, Cooper CS, Schmidt M, O'Brien SJ, Blair DG, and Vande Woude GF (1986) Mechanism of met oncogene activation. Cell 45, 895–904

Park M, Dean M, Kaul K, Braun MJ, Gonda MA, and Vande Woude G (1987) Sequence of MET protooncogene cDNA has features characteristic of the tyrosine kinase family of growth-factor receptors. Proc Natl Acad Sci U S A 84, 6379–6383

Peschard P, Fournier TM, Lamorte L, Naujokas MA, Band H, Langdon WY, and Park M (2001) Mutation of the c-Cbl TKB domain binding site on the Met receptor tyrosine kinase converts it into a transforming protein. Mol Cell 8, 995–1004

Peschard P, and Park M (2003) Escape from Cbl-mediated downregulation: a recurrent theme for oncogenic deregulation of receptor tyrosine kinases. Cancer Cell 3, 519–523

Petrelli A, Gilestro GF, Lanzardo S, Comoglio PM, Migone N, and Giordano S (2002) The endophilin-CIN85-Cbl complex mediates ligand-dependent downregulation of c-Met. Nature 416, 187–190

Ponzetto C, Bardelli A, Zhen Z, Maina F, dalla Zonca P, Giordano S, Graziani A, Panayotou G, and Comoglio PM (1994) A multifunctional docking site mediates signaling and transformation by the hepatocyte growth factor/scatter factor receptor family. Cell 77, 261–271

Potempa S, and Ridley AJ (1998) Activation of both MAP kinase and phosphatidylinositide 3-kinase by Ras is required for hepatocyte growth factor/scatter factor-induced adherens junction disassembly. Mol Biol Cell 9, 2185–2200

Raiborg C, Bache KG, Gillooly DJ, Madshus IH, Stang E, and Stenmark H (2002) Hrs sorts ubiquitinated proteins into clathrin-coated microdomains of early endosomes. Nat Cell Biol 4, 394–398

Ridley AJ, Comoglio PM, and Hall A (1995) Regulation of scatter factor/hepatocyte growth factor responses by Ras, Rac, and Rho in MDCK cells. Mol Cell Biol 15, 1110–1122

Rocca A, Lamaze C, Subtil A, and Dautry-Varsat A (2001) Involvement of the ubiquitin/proteasome system in sorting of the interleukin 2 receptor β chain to late endocytic compartments. Mol Biol Cell 12, 1293–1301

Rodrigues GA, and Park M (1993) Dimerization mediated through a leucine zipper activates the oncogenic potential of the met receptor tyrosine kinase. Mol Cell Biol 13, 6711–6722

Rodrigues GA, and Park M (1994) Oncogenic activation of tyrosine kinases. Curr Opin Genet Dev 4, 15–24

Rong S, Oskarsson M, Faletto D, Tsarfaty I, Resau JH, Nakamura T, Rosen E, Hopkins RF, and Vande Woude GF (1993) Tumorigenesis induced by co-expression of human hepatocyte growth factor and the human met proto-oncogene leads to high levels of expression of the ligand and the receptor. Cell Growth Differ 4, 563–594

Rubin JS, Chan AM, Bottaro DP, Burgess WH, Taylor WG, Cech AC, Hirschfield DW, Wong J, Miki T, Finch PW, and et al. (1991) A broad-spectrum human lung fibroblast-derived mitogen is a variant of hepatocyte growth factor. Proc Natl Acad Sci U S A 88, 415–419

Rusciano D, Lorenzoni P, and Burger MM (1996) Constitutive activation of c-Met in liver metastatic B16 melanoma cells depends on both substrate adhesion and cell density and is regulated by a cytosolic tyrosine phosphatase activity. J Biol Chem 271, 20763–20769

Russell WE, McGowan JA, and Bucher NL (1984a) Biological properties of a hepatocyte growth factor from rat platelets. J Cell Physiol 119, 193–197

Sachse M, Urbé S, Oorschot V, Strous GJ, and Klumperman J (2002) Bilayered clathrin coats on endosomal vacuoles are involved in protein sorting toward lysosomes. Mol Biol Cell 13, 1313–1328

Schaeper U, Gehring NH, Fuchs KP, Sachs M, Kempkes B, and Birchmeier W (2000) Coupling of Gab1 to c-Met, Grb2, and Shp2 mediates biological responses. J Cell Biol 149, 1419–1432

Schmidt A, Wolde M, Thiele C, Fest W, Kratzin H, Podtelejnikov AV, Witke W, Huttner WB, and Soling HD (1999) Endophilin I mediates synaptic vesicle formation by transfer of arachidonate to lysophosphatidic acid. Nature 401, 133–141

Schmidt L, Duh FM, Chen F, Kishida T, Glenn G, Choyke P, Scherer SW, Zhuang Z, Lubensky I, Dean M, et al. (1997) Germline and somatic mutations in the tyrosine kinase domain of the MET proto-oncogene in papillary renal carcinomas. Nat Genet 16, 68–73

Schnell JD, and Hicke L (2003) Non-traditional Functions of Ubiquitin and Ubiquitin-binding proteins. J Biol Chem

Sorkin A (1998) Endocytosis and intracellular sorting of receptor tyrosine kinases. Front Biosci 3, 729–738

Sorkin A, and von Zastrow M (2002) Signal transduction and endocytosis; close encounters of many kinds. Nature Rev Mol Cell Biol 3, 600–614

Soubeyran P, Kowanetz K, Szymkiewicz I, Langdon WY, and Dikic I (2002) Cbl-CIN85-endophilin complex mediates ligand-induced downregulation of EGF receptors. Nature 416, 183–187

Stoker M, Gherardi E, Perryman M, and Gray J (1987) Scatter factor is a fibroblast-derived modulator of epithelial cell mobility. Nature 327, 239–242

Tanimura S, Chatani Y, Hoshino R, Sato M, Watanabe S, Kataoka T, Nakamura T, and Kohno M (1998) Activation of the 41/43 kDa mitogen-activated protein kinase signaling pathway is required for hepatocyte growth factor-induced cell scattering. Oncogene 17, 57–65

Tebar F, Bohlander SK, and Sorkin A (1999) Clathrin assembly lymphoid myeloid leukemia (CALM) protein: localization in endocytic-coated pits, interactions with clathrin, and the impact of overexpression on clathrin-mediated traffic. Mol Biol Cell 10, 2687–2702

Thien CBF, Walker F, and Langdon WY (2001) Ring finger mutations that abolish c-Cbl directed polyubiquitination and down-regulation of the EGF receptor are insufficient for cell transformation. Mol Cell 7, 355–365

Trusolino L, Bertotti A, and Comoglio PM (2001) A signaling adapter function for $\alpha6\beta4$ integrin in the control of HGF-dependent invasive growth. Cell 107, 643–654

Trusolino L, and Comoglio PM (2002) Scatter-factor and semaphorin receptors: cell signalling for invasive growth. Nat Rev Cancer 2, 289–300

Urbé S, Mills IG, Stenmark H, Kitamura N, and Clague MJ (2000) Endosomal localization and receptor dynamics determine tyrosine phosphorylation of hepatocyte growth factor-regulated tyrosine kinase substrate. Mol Cell Biol 20, 7685–7692

van Kerkhof P, Govers R, Alves dos Santos CM, and Strous GJ (2000) Endocytosis and degradation of the growth hormone receptor are proteasome-dependent. J Biol Chem 275, 1575–1580

Vieria AV, Lamaze C, and Schmid SL (1996) Control of EGF receptor signaling by clathrin-mediated endocytosis. Science 274, 2086–2089

Villa-Moruzzi E, Puntoni F, Bardelli A, Vigna E, De Rosa S, and Comoglio PM (1998) Protein tyrosine phosphatase PTP-S binds to the juxtamembrane region of the hepatocyte growth factor receptor Met. Biochem J 336 (Pt 1), 235–239

Wechsler DS, Engstrom LD, Alexander BM, Motto DG, and Roulston D (2003) A novel chromosomal inversion at 11q23 in infant acute myeloid leukemia fuses MLL to CALM, a gene that encodes a clathrin assembly protein. Genes Chromosomes Cancer 36, 26–36

Weidner KM, Arakaki N, Hartmann G, Vandekerckhove J, Weingart S, Rieder H, Fonatsch C, Tsubouchi H, Hishida T, Daikuhara Y, et al. (1991) Evidence for the identity of human scatter factor and human hepatocyte growth factor. Proc Natl Acad Sci U S A 88, 7001–7005

Wells A, Welsh JB, Lazar CS, Wiley S, Gill GN, and Rosenfeld MG (1990) Ligand-induced transformation by a noninternalizing epidermal growth factor receptor. Science 247, 962–964

CTMI (2004) 286:45–79
© Springer-Verlag 2004

Signaling, Internalization, and Intracellular Activity of Fibroblast Growth Factor

A. Więdłocha (✉) · V. Sørensen

Department of Biochemistry, Institute for Cancer Research,
The Norwegian Radium Hospital, Montebello, 0310 Oslo, Norway
antoni.wiedlocha@labmed.uio.no

Abstract The fibroblast growth factor (FGF) family contains 23 members in mammals including its prototype members FGF-1 and FGF-2. FGFs have been implicated in regulation of many key cellular responses involved in developmental and physiological processes. These includes proliferation, differentiation, migration, apoptosis, angiogenesis, and wound healing. FGFs bind to five related, specific cell surface receptors (FGFRs). Four of these have intrinsic tyrosine kinase activity. Dimerization of the receptor is a prerequisite for receptor transphosphorylation and activation of downstream signaling molecules. All members of the FGF family have a high affinity for heparin and for cell surface heparan sulfate proteoglycans, which participate in formation of stable and active FGF-FGFR complexes. FGF-mediated signaling is an evolutionarily conserved signaling module operative in invertebrates and vertebrates. It seems that some members of the family have a dual mode of action. FGF-1, FGF-2, FGF-3, and FGF-11–14 have been found intranuclearly as endogenous proteins. Exogenous FGF-1 and FGF-2 are internalized by receptor-mediated endocytosis, in a clathrin-dependent and -independent way. Internalized FGF-1 and FGF-2 are able to cross cellular membranes to reach the cytosol and the nuclear compartment. The role of FGF internalization and the intracellular activity of some FGFs are discussed in the context of the known signaling induced by FGF.

1
The Fibroblast Growth Factor Family

The family of fibroblast growth factors (FGFs) currently consists of 23 structurally related polypeptides, including the two prototypes FGF-1 and -2 (Ornitz and Itoh 2001; Powers et al. 2000; Lander et al. 2001). Genes as well as transcripts and proteins of the family have also been identified in invertebrates. Two FGFs have been found in the roundworm *Caenorhabditis elegans* (Let-756 and Egl-17) (Burdine et al. 1997; Branda and Stern 2000; Borland et al. 2001), and a single *Fgf* gene (*branchless*), encoding an 84-kD polypeptide growth factor has been identified in *Drosophila* (Klambt et al. 1992; Ahmad and Baker 2002). Because the highest number of FGFs has been identified in vertebrates and because in the sea squirt *Ciona,* a basal chordate, six *Fgf* genes have been identified (Ornitz and Itoh 2001; Mason 2003), it seems that a process of evolutionary spreading out of the ancient *Fgf* gene(s) by duplication and divergence occurred early during chordate evolution (Coulier et al. 1997; Nagendra et al. 2001). This also reflects and stresses the crucial role of FGFs in vertebrate embryonic and fetal development (Szebenyi and Fallon 1999; Naski and Ornitz 1998; Vasiliauskas and Stern 2001; Bikfalvi et al. 1997).

In vertebrates the growth factors' molecular mass ranges from 17 to 34 kD. They share 13%–71% amino acid identity and contain a conserved 120-amino acid core region (Ornitz and Itoh 2001). The crystal structure of FGF-1 and -2 shows 12 antiparallel β strands arranged in a β-trefoil conformation (Zhang et al. 1991; Eriksson et al. 1991; Zhu et al. 1991; Pineda-Lucena et al. 1994; Blaber et al. 1996).

Additional diversity among members of the family is generated through the use of alternative translation initiation sites (FGF-2 and FGF-3) (Florkiewicz and Sommer 1989; Prats et al. 1989; Powell and Klagsbrun 1991; Acland et al. 1990) as well as by alternative splicing (avian FGF-2, FGF-5, FGF-8, FGF-11–14) (Zuniga Mejia et al. 1993; Munoz-Sanjuan et al. 2000; Ozawa et al. 1998; Tanaka et al. 1992; Munoz-Sanjuan et al. 1999; Wang et al. 2000).

Among the 23 identified members of the FGF family, FGF-1 and -2 are distinguished by the lack of a recognizable N-terminal signal sequence (Jaye et al. 1986; Abraham et al. 1986). After synthesis, these growth factors reside in the cytosol and/or nucleus of the producing cells (Sano et al. 1990; Cao et al. 1993). They are released from the cells by a mechanism bypassing the classic ER-Golgi secretory pathway (Mignatti et al. 1992; Mignatti and Rifkin 1991; Florkiewicz et al. 1995; Maciag and Friesel 1995; Cleves 1997; McNeil and Steinhardt 1997). Secretion of FGF-1 is increased under stress such as heat, hypoxia, or serum starvation (Jackson et al. 1995; Jackson et al. 1992; Mouta et al. 1998; Shin et al. 1996). Another leaderless subset of the FGF family (FGF-11–14) is believed not to be secreted at all and remains exclusively intracellular (Smallwood et al. 1996). Accumulating evidence indicates that FGF-1, FGF-2, and FGF-3 can act intracellularly as well as extracellularly (Imamura et al. 1990; Wiedlocha et al. 1994; Bouche et al. 1987; Stachowiak et al. 1994; Kiefer and Dickson 1995; Kiefer et al. 1994).

In cell culture FGFs can stimulate cell growth, migration, and differentiation. In vivo they are responsible for a wide spectrum of biological effects induced in different types of cells. The most important roles for FGF action are thought to be during development. The growth factors are expressed in a strict temporal and spatial pattern during embryonic differentiation and development of organs. In brief, they are involved in development of the skeleton, limbs, and circulatory and central nervous systems (Goldfarb 1996; Ciruna and Rossant 2001; Celli et al. 1998; Martin 1998; Vasiliauskas and Stern 2001). In an adult organism FGFs are involved in wound healing, tissue repair, angiogenesis (FGF-1, -2), and mechanisms involved in homeostatic regulations (Burgess and Maciag 1989; Rieck et al. 1992; Werner et al. 1992; Friesel and Maciag 1995). Members of the family have also been recognized as factors involved in some pathological conditions, particularly neoplasia (Wright and Huang 1996; Halaban 1996), diabetic retinopathy, and atherosclerosis (Brogi et al. 1993; Cuevas et al. 1991; Liau et al. 1993; Hughes 1996).

The biological action of FGFs is exerted through binding to and activation of high-affinity cell surface FGF receptors (FGFRs) that have intrinsic tyrosine kinase activity (Schlessinger 2000). Additionally, all recognized members of the FGF family contain a heparin and heparan sulfate-binding domain. Binding of the growth factors to heparan sulfate proteoglycans (HSPGs) present at the cell surface and in the extracellular matrix protects them against proteases and thermal denaturation (Copeland et al. 1991) and regulates binding to and activation of FGFRs (Rapraeger et al. 1991). It also creates a local reservoir of FGFs (Ruoslahti and Yamaguchi 1991).

2
The Cell Surface Binding Sites

2.1
The Family of FGF Receptors

The FGFR family contains five closely related genes. At least three of these encode multiple receptor isoforms. FGFR1–4 have a conserved overall structure composed of three extracellular Ig-like domains (D1–

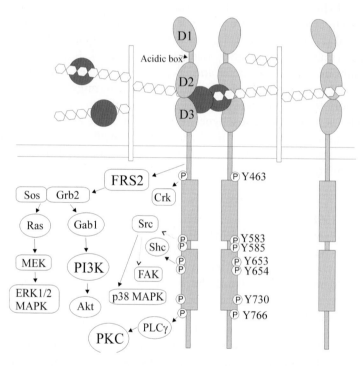

Fig. 1. Illustration of the FGFR structure, binding of FGF to FGFR, and the intracellular signaling pathways activated by FGF/FGFR. FGFR (*gray*) consists of three Ig-like extracellular domains (*D1–3*), an "acidic box," a transmembrane region, and an intracellular region confining a split tyrosine kinase domain (*boxes*). FGF (*black circles*) binds to the carbohydrate moieties (heparans) of HSPG (*white*) and to the FGFR in the D2–D3 region. Also, FGFR contains a heparan binding site in D2. The ternary active receptor complex is believed to consist of FGF, FGFR, and heparan with a 2:2:2 stoichiometry, where heparan is buried between the two FGF-molecules but also touches FGFR in D2. The seven tyrosine phosphorylation sites identified in FGFR1 are indicated. *Arrows* indicate interactions/activations of downstream adaptor or signaling molecules as illustrated

D3), a unique acidic region (acidic box), a transmembrane domain, and a well-conserved split tyrosine kinase domain (Fig. 1). They share up to 70% identity (Powers et al. 2000; Burke et al. 1998). The fifth member of the gene family does not contain a tyrosine kinase domain but still has 32% identity with the other FGF receptors within the extracellular part (Sleeman et al. 2001). Additional diversity among members of the family is generated by mechanisms based on alternative splicing of FGFR mRNA and alternative promoter activity resulting in receptor isoforms (Johnson and Williams 1993; Johnson et al. 1991; Johnson et al. 1990; Goldstrohm et al. 2001; Yan et al. 1993). This can result in expression of soluble extracellular forms (Hanneken et al. 1994; Hanneken et al. 1995; Guillonneau et al. 1998; Celli et al. 1998; Jang 2002), variants devoid of the tyrosine kinase domain (Ueno et al. 1992; Li et al. 1994; van Heumen et al. 1999), or variants with distinct ligand binding specificities (Yu and Ornitz 2001; Yeh et al. 2003). Even intracellular isoforms of the receptor can be generated (Johnston et al. 1995; Ezzat et al. 2002). Genes of the FGFR family are well conserved throughout vertebrate evolution (Goldfarb 1996). Each of the receptors binds more than one member of the FGF family with high affinity.

2.2
Heparan Sulfate Proteoglycans

Proteoglycans are complex structures located predominantly on the cell surface and in the extracellular matrix (Ruoslahti and Yamaguchi 1991). They consist of a core protein and several carbohydrate moieties. The core protein can be transmembrane, or it can be linked to the membrane by a glycosylphosphatidylinositol (GPI) anchor. The carbohydrate moieties (glycosaminoglycans) are polymers of disaccharide repeats, which are mostly highly sulfated and negatively charged. The main glycosaminoglycans in proteoglycans are chondroitin sulfate, dermatan sulfate, heparan sulfate, heparin, and keratin sulfate. Heparan sulfate contains low and highly sulfated sites, whereas heparin is more uniformly highly sulfated (Galzie et al. 1997). Heparan sulfate proteoglycans (HSPGs) serve as low-affinity FGF cell surface receptors (Fig. 1).

2.3
Cysteine-Rich FGF Receptor

Various FGFs bind with high affinity also to a cysteine-rich FGF receptor (CFR) without tyrosine kinase activity (Burrus and Olwin 1989; Burrus et al. 1992; Zhou et al. 1997). This type of receptor does not belong to the FGFR family, and its function is generally unknown, although there are reports indicating that it is involved in intracellular regulation of FGF secretion (Zuber et al. 1997; Kohl et al. 2000). CFR binds FGF-1–4 in a heparin-independent manner but exhibits high affinity for HSPGs (Zhou et al. 1997). CFR is a transmembrane sialoglycoprotein primarily located in the Golgi apparatus, whereas its proteolytic cleavage fragment has also been found secreted and deposited in the extracellular matrix (Gonatas et al. 1995). The amino acid sequence of the receptor shows 16 cysteine-rich repeats in the intraluminar domain and a short cytoplasmic tail (Mourelatos et al. 1996).

A protein with high sequence similarity (possibly identical) to the CFR, containing a 70-amino acid N-terminal extension, was shown to be a ligand for the cell adhesion molecule E-selectin (Steegmaier et al. 1995).

2.4
Binding of FGF to High-Affinity Tyrosine Kinase Receptor

Most FGFs can bind to and activate more than one FGFR. FGFR1–4 have different specificities for different FGFs. Additional specificity of ligand binding to FGFR1–3 is determined by alternative splicing of exons in the region encoding the growth factor binding subdomain (exons IIIa, IIIb, or IIIc of D3). Such alternative splicing events are regulated in a tissue-specific manner. Usually, the expression of IIIb is restricted to epithelial cells and IIIc to mesenchymal cells (Goldstrohm et al. 2001; Beer et al. 2000; Orr-Urtreger et al. 1993).

Binding of the FGF ligand to its specific FGFR results in receptor dimerization and autophosphorylation at tyrosine residues in the intracellular part of the receptor. Ligand-induced dimerization is a key event that leads to an increase in the kinase activity of the receptor (Schlessinger 2000). It should be kept in mind that binding to and dimerization of the specific tyrosine kinase receptor by FGF is a more complex process than in the case of other growth factors. In contrast to EGF or PDGF, which simply bridge two receptor molecules (Heldin and Ostman 1996), FGF alone apparently cannot induce formation of stable receptor dimers but requires HSPG/heparin (Spivak-Kroizman et al. 1994). A dual-receptor model for FGF is based on the interaction of growth factor with both HSPG/heparin and the tyrosin kinase receptor (Rapraeger et al. 1991; Yayon et al. 1991; Klagsbrun and Baird 1991; Ornitz et al. 1992; Spivak-Kroizman et al. 1994). It was proposed that cell surface HSPGs form oligomeric complexes with FGF able to bind to a few FGFRs, leading to assembly of active FGF-FGFR dimers. Several reports describing the crystal structure of FGF-1 or -2 in complex with FGFR1 or -2 have been published (Plotnikov et al. 2000; Plotnikov et al. 1999; Stauber et al. 2000; Pellegrini et al. 2000; Schlessinger et al. 2000). The emerging picture is that FGF binds FGFR in the D2-D3 junction and that heparin is involved in bridging and stabilizing two FGF-FGFR complexes in a receptor-dimer complex (Fig. 1).

Several more recent reports have shown that FGF can also activate FGFR in the absence of HSPGs (Fannon and Nugent 1996; Lin et al. 1999; Delehedde et al. 2000; Lundin et al. 2003; Lundin et al. 2000), although HSPGs generally are required for formation of stable FGF-FGFR signaling complexes. *Drosophila* lacking enzymes for sulfation of glycosaminoglycans was found to have a phenotype similar to those lacking fibroblast growth factor receptors, but the requirement for heparan sulfate could partially be overcome by overexpression of the *Drosophila* FGF homolog, *Branchless* (Lin et al. 1999). This proves a crucial role for sulfated heparans in FGF signaling and indicates that two forms of the growth factor-receptor signaling complex can exist, a less stable FGF-FGFR complex and a more stable ternary structure of FGF-FGFR-HSPG with prolonged signaling activity (Ornitz 2000).

It has been shown that the pattern of sulfation of heparan sulfates correlates with FGFR activation (Lundin et al. 2000). Furthermore, it was suggested, based on in vitro modification of HSPGs and a cell genetic study, that different binding sites on sulfated heparans in HSPGs are involved in the FGF-1 and FGFR binding and in the ternary complex formation (Wu et al. 2003). On the basis of these studies a model of 2:2:2 stoichiometry of FGF-1-heparan-FGFR was proposed.

In vitro, FGF-1-induced stimulation of DNA synthesis in mouse fibroblasts requires continuous treatment with the growth factor for as much as 12 h (Zhan et al. 1993). This is consistent with the requirement for stable FGF-FGFR-HSPG complex formation to induce a mitogenic signal.

FGFRs also contain a heparin-binding site in D2 that is involved in formation of the signaling complex (Wu et al. 2003; Kan et al. 1993). Therefore, it is not excluded that heparans as such could induce FGFR dimerization and activation without the growth factor (Gao and Goldfarb 1995; Sakaguchi et al. 1999). To protect against this, it was proposed that the acidic box between D1 and D2 interacts with a basic subdomain in D2 competing for binding to HSPGs (Schlessinger 2003). In this way,

D1 and the acidic box might play an autoinhibitory role, regulating binding of heparans and FGF to FGFR.

3
FGF Receptor Signaling

In the case of FGFR1, the most widely expressed and best-characterized FGF receptor, seven phosphotyrosines have been identified as binding sides for downstream signaling molecules containing SH2 domains (Klint and Claesson-Welsh 1999). It has been shown that PLCγ_1 (Burgess et al. 1990; Mohammadi et al. 1991) and the adapter molecules Shc, Crk, Shb, and FGF receptor substrate 2 (FRS2) (Klint et al. 1995; Larsson et al. 1999; Cross et al. 2002; Kouhara et al. 1997) bind directly to activated FGFR1. FRS2 binds to the receptor in a phosphotyrosine-independent manner (Ong et al. 2000). During receptor activation FRS2 is phosphorylated at multiple tyrosine residues, providing new binding sides for direct or indirect recruitment of multiprotein complexes that are responsible for both activation and attenuation of signaling (Ong et al. 2000; Wong et al. 2002; Lax et al. 2002). It appears that PLC-γ/protein kinase (PK)C, PI3K/Akt, and Ras/MAPK are three major downstream signaling pathways activated by FGFs (Boilly et al. 2000) (Fig. 1). Grb2 binds to a phosphotyrosine of FRS2, recruits SOS to the plasma membrane, and activates the Ras pathway (Klint and Claesson-Welsh 1999). PI3K appears to be directly bound to Gab1, which is recruited by Grb2 to the FRS2-receptor complex as well (Ong et al. 2001). Moreover, it was reported that FRS2 could link FGFR activation to atypical PKC isoforms (Lim et al. 1999).

It has been shown that PKA is able to control the activation and duration of the growth factor-stimulated Ras/ERK pathway (Yao et al. 1998; Pursiheimo et al. 2002a). FGF-2 was shown to stimulate the activity of PKA, and it was shown that activation of a FGF-inducible response element on the syndecan-1 gene by FGF-2 requires the cooperational function of PKA and the Ras/ERK pathway (Pursiheimo et al. 2002b; Pursiheimo et al. 2000).

When Grb2 is bound to Spry1 and Spry2, which are translocated to the plasma membrane and become phosphorylated after FGF stimulation, the recruitment of Grb2-SOS to FRS2 is inhibited (Hanafusa et al. 2002). Recently, the transmembrane protein Sef was also found to inhibit FGF induced proliferation by interaction with FGFR (Kovalenko et al. 2003).

It was also shown that a serine kinase (p85) is associated with activated FGFR4, implicating a role for serine phosphorylation in signal transmission by the receptor (Vainikka et al. 1996).

FGFR1 can stimulate or inhibit Src kinase activity in a PKC-dependent manner (Klint and Claesson-Welsh 1999). Although there are conflicting reports concerning direct binding of Src to FGFR1 (Zhan et al. 1994; Landgren et al. 1995), it is accepted that the kinase is involved in a variety of signaling cascades in FGF-stimulated cells (Yayon et al. 1997). Similarly to Src, another cytoplasmic tyrosine kinase, FAK, is activated under FGF stimuli as well as in response to extracellular matrix-mediated ligation of integrins. Because focal adhesions contain FGF receptor, it appears that at least part of the receptor-induced signaling, including activation of Src and FAK, can be involved in integrin-mediated signal transduction (Plopper et al. 1995).

Interestingly, FGF-1 induces biphasic tyrosine phosphorylation events and the maximum level of FGF-1-induced DNA synthesis requires the continued presence of growth factor for at least 12 h (Zhan et al. 1993; Imamura et al. 1994). There is also a report demonstrating that, in vitro, a transient stimulation of mouse fibroblasts with FGF-1 was sufficient for sustained activation of Src and thereby induction of a migrating phenotype. On the other hand, only long-term stimulation with FGF-1 led to sustained activation of Erk1 and Erk2 kinases, and this correlated with cell proliferation (LaVallee et al. 1998). Phosphorylation of cortactin, the F-actin binding protein, by Src is an important part of the migratory response. This indicates that FGF-1 stimuli can be dissociated into signals more specific for cell migration via Src and p38 MAP kinase and signals able to induce cell proliferation through Erk kinase (Boilly et al. 2000; Liu et al. 1999).

It has also been shown that FGF-2 transduces different signals through FGFR-1 depending on the presence or absence of heparin/HSPG. In the absence of heparin, FGF-2 was found to induce increased phosphorylation of Tyr463 of FGFR-1 and maximal phosphorylation of the phosphatase SHP-2 and Crk, whereas heparin had to be present to achieve maximal phosphorylation of Tyr766 of FGFR-1 and Shb and PLCγ (Lundin et al. 2003).

It should be noted that cell adhesion molecules like N-CAM and C-cadherin interact with FGFR and induce FGFR-mediated signaling in an FGF-independent manner (Cavallaro et al. 2001). With a recently developed experimental system, it was reported that activation of an engineered FGFR1 that can be induced to dimerize by the drug AP20187 resulted in alterations in cell polarity and hyperproliferation of epithelial cells in mammary glands of transgenic mice (Welm et al. 2002).

Recently, it was reported that the HSPG syndecan-4 core protein, which binds PIP_2 and activates $PKC\alpha$, participates in mediating effects in response to FGF-2 stimulation (Horowitz et al. 2002). Mutations in the intracellular part of syndecan-4 that either decreased its affinity to PIP_2 or disrupted its PDZ-dependent binding resulted in its hyperphosphorylation after FGF stimulation, and this was reflected in a reduced ability of endothelial cells to respond to FGF-2 stimuli. This suggests that $PKC\alpha$ activation and PDZ-dependent formation of a phosphatase-containing complex by syndecan-4 is a significant part of the signaling events induced by FGF-2. It also indicates that HSPGs can directly participate in downstream events of FGF/FGFR signaling and not only in the FGF-FGFR complex formation.

It has been shown that certain mutations in FGFR1, -2, and -3 provoke skeletal disorders like achondroplasia, hypochondrioplasia, or Crouzon syndrome (Shiang et al. 1994; De Moerlooze and Dickson 1997). Although the mutations are localized in the extracellular domain as well as in the intracellular part of the receptors (Ornitz and Marie 2002; Burke et al. 1998), it appears that they are involved in a common molecular basis for those syndromes, a constitutively active, ligand-independent dimer of the receptor.

4
Endocytosis and Intracellular Sorting of the FGF-FGFR Complex

After binding to its high-affinity receptor, FGF is rapidly internalized (Marchese et al. 1998; Roghani and Moscatelli 1992; Sorokin et al. 1994; Fannon and Nugent 1996; Friesel and Maciag 1988). The endocytic pathway taken by FGF/FGFR has been addressed in only a few studies. It appears that the different FGFR isoforms use different pathways, and this seems to vary also between different cell types.

Several reports have shown that FGF/FGFRs are taken up by the clathrin-mediated pathway. KGF/KGFR (i.e., FGF-7 and a splice variant of FGFR2) was reported to be internalized through clathrin-coated pits in NIH/3T3 cells stably transfected with KGFR, as well as in A253 carcinoma cells and in human cultured keratinocytes (Marchese et al. 1998). It was also found that mitogenesis in NIH/3T3 cells stimulated by FGF-1 was inhibited by inhibition of clathrin-mediated endocytosis (Grieb and Burgess 2000). Also, FGF-1/FGFR4 was found to be endocytosed partly by a clathrin-dependent pathway in FGFR4-transfected HeLa cells (Citores et al. 2001).

In contrast to this, FGF-2 was reported to be endocytosed mainly through caveolae in BHK cells and ABAE cells (Gleizes et al. 1996). Furthermore, FGF-1/FGFR4 was reported to be endocytosed mainly by a mechanism different from the clathrin-mediated pathway and caveolae in COS cells and also partly by a nonclathrin/noncaveolae mechanism in HeLa cells (Citores et al. 2001; Citores et al. 1999).

The signals within the FGFR that mediate endocytosis are not very well defined, but phosphorylation events induced by the receptor tyrosine kinase appear to play a role for efficient endocytosis. A decreased internalization of FGFR1 was observed by mutation of the major autophosphorylation site 766 and for a kinase-dead FGFR1 (Sorokin et al. 1994). The phosphotyrosine in position 766 is the binding site for PLCγ. A decrease in endocytosis was also observed for FGFR4 when it lacked the region encompassing the C-terminal phosphorylation site (Munoz et al. 1997) or when the kinase domain was inactive or deleted (Citores et al. 2001). However, in neither of these cases was internalization completely blocked, suggesting that other endocytosis signals independent of the kinase domain exist in the FGFR. Consistently, a more drastic reduction in the endocytosis of FGFR4 was observed when almost the entire cytosolic region of FGFR4 was deleted (Citores et al. 2001).

After their internalization from the plasma membrane, FGF-FGFR complexes enter early sorting endosomes (Citores et al. 1999; Gleizes et al. 1996), as is expected for internalized receptors irrespective of their mechanism of internalization (van Deurs et al. 1989). Subsequent to their presence in early endosomes, KGF/KGFR was found to be sorted to late endosomes (Belleudi et al. 2002). Also, FGF-2 was found to be sorted to late endosomes and lysosomes in BHK cells (Gleizes et al. 1996). On the other hand, FGF-1/FGFR4 was sorted mainly to the perinuclear recycling compartment in COS cells and in HeLa cells (Citores et al. 1999). This sorting was apparently regulated by the receptor kinase, because a kinase-dead mutant of FGFR4 showed increased transport to lysosomes (Citores et al. 2001).

FGF can be internalized also by binding to surface HSPGs (Roghani and Moscatelli 1992). FGF-1 and FGF-2 internalized by binding to HSPGs were shown to be sorted to lysosomes (Gleizes et al. 1995; Citores et al. 2001).

Consistent with the current knowledge that signaling from receptor molecules occurs not only at the plasma membrane but also from internalized ligand-receptor complexes, KGF and KGFR were found to remain associated in active complexes through the endocytic pathway (Belleudi et al. 2002; Marchese et al. 1998) and activated FGFR4 was found in the recycling endosomal compartment (Citores et al. 1999).

Internalized FGF is unusually long lived (Bikfalvi et al. 1989; Bouche et al. 1987; Moenner et al. 1989; Moscatelli 1988). In various cell types only 10%–30% of the internalized FGF was found to be degraded after 6–8 h (Munoz et al. 1997; Citores et al. 2001), and FGF can be detected as late as 24 h after internalization (Friesel and Maciag 1988; Grieb and Burgess 2000).

FGFR internalization leads to desensitization, and degradation of the receptor has been detected after a few hours (Sorokin et al. 1994; Belleudi et al. 2002; Bikfalvi et al. 1989; Moscatelli and Devesly 1990). It has been shown that binding of FGF induces ubiquitination of FGFR1 and FGFR3, and this contributes to receptor downregulation (Mori et al. 1995; Wong et al. 2002; Monsonego-Ornan et al. 2002). FGFR was found to recruit the ubiquitin ligase Cbl by an indirect mechanism involving the docking protein FRS2α and Grb2 (Wong et al. 2002).

It has been reported that FGF-2 stimulation induces nuclear transcellocation of FGFR1 (Maher 1996). The nuclear import of FGFR1 was found to be mediated by importin β and was found to play a role in the regulation of the cell cycle (Reilly and Maher 2001). FGFR1 thus is one of many transmembrane receptors that have been demonstrated to also have a nuclear localization (Jans and Hassan 1998; Goldfarb 2001). It has been suggested that the association of the FGFR1 transmembrane region with the ER membrane is relatively unstable and that the nucleus-destined receptor is released from the ER/Golgi membranes into the cytosol before delivery to the plasma membrane (Myers et al. 2003).

5
Intracellular Localization of Exogenous FGF

Protein hormones, growth factors, and cytokines have been recognized as regulatory agents operating at the cell surface before internalization into endosomal vesicles, where they induce signaling as long as they are not degraded in lysosomal compartments. According to this view, during the period of their action the growth factors should always be separated from the cytosol by a membrane.

In the case of certain FGFs the nature of signals responsible for FGF-mediated biological effects seems to be more complex. Evidence for cell entry of exogenous FGF-1 and -2 has been accumulating over the last decade (Olsnes et al. 2003).

Not only does FGF-1 activate the cell surface receptor, but the receptor-bound growth factor is also endocytosed and translocated across the membrane (Wiedlocha et al. 1995; Klingenberg et al. 1998) to reach the cytosol and the nucleus. Nuclear localization appears to depend on the presence of a nuclear localization sequence (NLS) in FGF-1 (Imamura et al. 1990; Imamura et al. 1994; Friedman et al. 1994; Wiedlocha et al. 1994). It was shown that removal of the NLS prevents translocation to the nucleus and also stimulation of DNA synthesis, but not tyrosine phosphorylation and c-fos induction. The mitogenic activity was recovered when an NLS from yeast histone was inserted into the growth factor mutant (Imamura et al. 1990).This suggests that exogenous FGF enters the nucleus ,where it stimulates DNA synthesis. However, one should take into consideration the fact that the FGF-1 NLS mutant has reduced affinity for heparin and is therefore more sensitive for proteolytic degradation. Therefore, the mutated growth factor might not form stable complexes with the receptor and will therefore induce transient and weaker signaling. On the other hand, a correlation between stimulation of DNA synthesis and transport of radiolabeled FGF-1 to the nuclear fraction has been demonstrated, and it occurs during the entire G_1 phase of the cell cycle (Zhan et al. 1993; Imamura et al. 1994).

Further evidence for membrane translocation of externally added FGF-1 was obtained by treatment of FGFR-positive cells with a growth factor mutant containing a C-terminal farnesylation signal, a CAAX-box. Because the farnesyl transferase is located exclusively in the cytosol and nucleus (Clarke 1992), the appearance of farnesylated FGF-1-CAAX indicated that the growth factor had crossed cellular membranes (Wiedlocha et al. 1995). Another method used to assess membrane translocation takes advantage of the fact that FGF-1 has a functional phosphorylation site (S130) and that it is phosphorylated by PKC, an enzyme that is also exclusively present in the cytosol and nucleus. Phosphorylation of externally added growth factor at this site indicated that FGF-1 had translocated into the cytosol and/or nucleus (Klingenberg et al. 1998). It has been shown that translocation of exogenous FGF-1 to the cytosol and nucleus requires binding to FGFR (Wiedlocha et al. 1995; Klingenberg et al. 1998; Klingenberg et al. 2000a). Although the growth factor also binds abundantly to HSPGs, in cells lacking FGFRs the FGF-1 was not translocated to the cytosol and nucleus (Klingenberg et al. 1998), indicating that FGFR plays a crucial role in this process.

With the use of farnesylation and phosphorylation approaches to study translocation of FGF-1 into cells it was found that full-length FGFR4, with an active or inactive kinase domain, facilitated transloca-tion of the growth factor to the cytosol and nucleus. Also, a receptor mutant with deletion of the kinase domain was able to mediate translo-cation of exogenous FGF-1 to the cytosol. In contrast, a mutant of FGFR4 with deletion of only the last 11 amino acids in the cytosolic do-main did not support translocation of FGF-1 into cells (Klingenberg et al. 2000a). This points out the extreme C-terminus of FGFR4 as an im-portant determinant for translocation of FGF-1 to the cytosol and nucle-us.

The transport of FGF-1 to the cytosol and the nucleus depends on signaling mechanisms in the cytosol. PI3K seems to be involved in this process because inhibitors of this enzyme, wortmannin and LY294002, prevent translocation of the growth factor into the cell interior (Klingen-berg et al. 2000b). A tyrosine kinase inhibitor, genistein, inhibits the translocation of FGF-1 into cells as well (Munoz et al. 1997). Recently obtained data have shown that translocation of the growth factor to the cytosol occurs from the lumen of intracellular vesicles possessing vacuo-lar proton pumps and that an electrical potential across the vesicular membrane, generated by these pumps, is required for FGF-1 transloca-tion (Malecki et al. 2002). Inhibition of endosomal acidification by am-monium chloride or monensin did not block the translocation process, whereas bafilomycin A1 or concanamycin A, specific inhibitors of vacu-olar proton pumps, blocked translocation completely. When the polar-ization of the vesicular membrane was regenerated by activation of Na^+/K^+-ATPase in the membrane, the growth factor was again able to trans-locate to the cytosol.

Translocation of proteins across membranes usually requires a cer-tain extent of unfolding. However, FGF-1 disulfide-bonded mutants and an irreversibly cross-linked mutant that remains in a folded state were translocated to the cytosol and the nucleus equally well as wild-type FGF-1 (Wesche et al. 2000). Because transport of proteins to peroxi-somes and into the thylakoid membrane of chloroplasts also does not re-quire extensive unfolding, the translocation of FGF-1 into cells in a fold-ed state is not unique.

FGF-1 fused to the N-terminus of diphtheria toxin could be translo-cated as a passenger protein, via the toxin entry road, into cells lacking receptors for the growth factor. With the use of cells that were mutated to be resistant to the intracellular action of the toxin, it could be demon-strated that the fusion protein was translocated to the cytosol and then subsequently to the nucleus, in a growth factor NLS-dependent manner. Finally, stimulation of DNA synthesis was induced only when the full-length fusion protein (translocation competent) containing wild-type FGF-1 was given to the cells lacking FGFR (Wiedlocha et al. 1994). Despite this, there was no proliferation of the cells. In further experiments it was demonstrated that the presence and activation of FGFR was also necessary to induce cell proliferation (Wiedlocha et al. 1996).

Also, in the case of FGF-2, several authors have reported transport of the exogenous growth factor to the nucleus. It was shown that FGF-2 accumulated in the nucleus and nucleoli during the G_1 stage and that this correlated with the stimulation of ribosomal gene transcription (Bouche et al. 1987) and cellular proliferation (Baldin et al. 1990; Bonnet et al. 1996). The growth factor was also reported to be able to stimulate transcription in a cell-free system (Nakanishi et al. 1992).

6
Intracellular Localization of Endogenous FGF

Although most FGFs contain a leader sequence for efficient secretion from cells, a few members of the family have been found to accumulate in the cytosol and/or nucleus of cells producing them (Cao et al. 1993; Prudovsky et al. 2002). FGF-1 is synthesized as one isoform usually detected in the cytoplasm; however, the endogenous, intracellular growth factor can also accumulate in the nuclear compartment. It was found that FGF-1 localized to the nuclei of cells in inflammatory arthritic joints (Sano et al. 1990). When overexpressed in cells, FGF was found to accumulate in nuclei (Cao et al. 1993). Moreover, it was demonstrated that nuclear accumulation of the growth factor depends on an N-terminally located basic amino acid sequence that can serve as an NLS (Imamura et al. 1990; Imamura et al. 1992; Friedman et al. 1994).

Efficient export of FGF-1 from cells is observed under stress conditions. The cytoplasmic domain of synaptotagmin (Tarantini et al. 1998) and the calcium binding protein S100A13 (Mouta et al. 1998) are involved in the FGF-1 nonclassic release process (Cleves 1997). It has been demonstrated that before FGF-1 release, both synaptotagmin and S100A13 colocalize with the growth factor near the inner surface of the plasma membrane. Formation of this intracellular complex appears to be dependent on F-actin (Prudovsky et al. 2002). It has also been shown that the partially unfolded conformation of FGF-1 disrupts the membrane integrity of negatively charged liposomes (Mach and Middaugh 1995) and that FGF-1 is secreted as a homodimer (Tarantini et al. 1998).

FGF-2 is synthesized as five isoforms (18, 22, 22.5, 24, and 34 kD). It was found that these isoforms are associated with different intracellular complexes (Patry et al. 1997). The high-molecular-mass isoforms are generated by alternative initiation of translation, at CUG initiation sites upstream, in-frame of the Kozak AUG methionine codon (Bugler et al. 1991; Vagner et al. 1995). Only the 18-kD isoform, which is translated from AUG, is primarily cytosolic, and it is released by a mechanism sensitive to drugs like probenicid (Gupta et al. 1998) and ouabain (Dahl et al. 2000; Florkiewicz et al. 1998). This suggests that multidrug resistance-associated proteins and the Na^+/K^+-ATPase are involved in the cell release process. It was also shown that a 27-kD heat shock protein facilitates the 18-kD FGF-2 export (Piotrowicz et al. 1997). The high-molecular-mass isoforms of FGF-2 are detectable exclusively in the nucleus as endogenous proteins. They contain in the N-terminal extensions several GR repeats that act as NLS. Although the intracellular role of the high-molecular-mass isoforms is still not well known, there are reports indicating that they might have an intracrine, perhaps nuclear, function, because they are able to stimulate cell growth under low-serum conditions (Bikfalvi et al. 1995; Vagner et al. 1996; Arese et al. 1999). Furthermore, intravenous injection of bladder carcinoma cells producing 24-kD FGF-2 into nude mice led to extensive lung metastasis, whereas injection of cells producing 18-kD FGF-2, or not producing any isoform of the growth factor, did not induce metastasis (Okada-Ban et al. 1999). Also, it was reported that the intracellular high-molecular-mass isoforms of FGF-2 cause transdifferentiation of avian neural crest-derived Schwann cell precursors into melanocytes (Sherman et al. 1993). The distribution of FGF-2 between nucleus and cytosol was observed during early development (Riese et al. 1995).

It was found that the level of intracellular 18-, 22-, and 24-kD FGF-2 isoforms in adrenal chromaffin cells could be increased by stimulation of acetylcholine receptors or angiotensin II receptors or by direct stimulation of adenylate cyclase or PKC (Stachowiak et al. 1994). The increased level of the growth factor isoforms was observed in the cytosol and the nucleus but not in the extracellular medium. It was shown that FGF-2 acts as an intracrine nuclear growth factor with putative function as a regulator of genomic responses to afferent stimulation of adrenal medullary cells. In a subsequent report it was shown that translocation of FGF-2 from the cytosol to the nucleus correlated with proliferation in normal astrocytes, whereas contact inhibition between cells was associated with redistribution of the growth factor to the cytosol. On the other hand, FGF-2 was constitutively nuclear in glioblastoma cells (Joy et al. 1997).

The recently described 34-kD isoform of FGF-2 contains an arginine-rich NLS in the N-terminal region similar to the NLS of HIV type 1 Rev and Tat proteins. Expression of the 34-kD isoform permitted mouse fibroblast survival in low-serum conditions (Arnaud et al. 1999).

In the case of FGF-3, intracellular localization is determined by an NLS, competing with an N-terminal leader sequence (Kiefer et al. 1994; Antoine et al. 1997). Therefore, the growth factor can be secreted by the classic ER-Golgi pathway and through binding to FGFR stimulate cell growth. On the other hand, it can also be nuclear and inhibit cell proliferation through a not well-known mechanism (Kiefer and Dickson 1995).

FGF-9 lacks an N-teminal signal sequence. Instead, the growth factor contains a noncleaved hydrophobic region in the center of the molecule that is required for secretion through the ER and Golgi complex (Miyamoto et al. 1993). Also, FGF-16 and -20, which are homologs of FGF-9, do not have a classic signal sequence (Miyake et al. 1998; Ohmachi et al. 2000).

A distinct branch (subfamily) in the FGF family consists of FGF-11–14, also referred to as the FGF homology factors (FHFs) (Smallwood et al. 1996; Munoz-Sanjuan et al. 1999). They share less than 30% amino acid identity with other FGFs but up to 70% identity among themselves. None of them contains a signal sequence, but all have basic residues resembling an NLS. It was shown that FGF-11 accumulates in the nucleus in an NLS-dependent manner (Smallwood et al. 1996). FHFs are not secreted and remain intracellular when transfected into different cell lines (Smallwood et al. 1996; Wang et al. 2000). It was reported that they can bind heparin with high affinity like other FGFs, but they are not able to activate any of the FGFRs (Olsen et al. 2003). These FGFs were found to be expressed mainly in the developing and adult nervous system.

7
Molecular Targets of Intracellular FGF

Although the extracellular action of FGF is understood in some detail, the intracellular trafficking of some FGFs, as well as their mode of intracellular action, remains largely unexplained. To find out more, different approaches like pull-down experiments (Skjerpen et al. 2002b), coimmunoprecipitation (Mizukoshi et al. 1999), the yeast two-hybrid system (Kolpakova et al. 1998; Mizukoshi et al. 1999; Van den et al. 2000; Reimers et al. 2001), in vivo colocalization (Skjerpen et al. 2002a; Mizukoshi et al. 1999), and an in vivo protein-protein interaction assay (Skjerpen et al. 2002a) have been applied. It should be kept in mind that by using these methods it is difficult to distinguish exogenous FGF from endogenous, intracellular FGF. It is not excluded that intracellular mechanisms of action of endogenous and exogenous growth factors are different, because the cell entry of exogenous growth factor requires binding to FGFR. This induces a signaling cascade that might activate regulatory pathways distinct from those of resting cells.

Intracellular FGF presumably interacts with other proteins that are involved in trafficking and functioning of the growth factor. An interaction between FGF-1 and FGF-1 intracellular binding protein (FIBP) was identified by a yeast two-hybrid screen. FIBP is located on the cytosolic side of ER, on the outer mitochondrial membrane, and inside the nucleus, and it is abundantly and widely expressed in mammalian tissue and cultured cells (Kolpakova et al. 1998). FIBP mRNA is present as early as the blastocyst stage in mice. However, the exact biological function of FIBP remains to be elucidated.

Another intracellular protein able to interact with FGF-1 is mortalin/GRP75, a member of the hsp70 family of heat shock proteins, also recognized as regulators of glucose responses, antigen processing, and cell mortality (Mizukoshi et al. 1999). FGF-1-mortalin interaction was shown to occur in vivo by coimmunoprecipitation and immunohistochemical colocalization methods, and by the yeast two-hybrid system, and also in vitro by a binding assay using recombinant FGF-1.

CK2 has been identified as a protein able to bind to FGF-1 via the catalytic α-subunit as well as the regulatory β-subunit. With a novel method assaying for intracellular protein-protein interactions (Skjerpen et al. 2002a), it was shown that FGF-1 and CK2 interact in vivo. In the same study it was found that in vitro, the growth factor is phosphorylated by CK2, and the presence of FGF-1 was found to enhance the autophosphorylation of CK2β. Moreover, a correlation between the mitogenic potential of a series of FGF-1 mutants and their ability to bind to CK2α was observed (Skjerpen et al. 2002a).

Ribosome-binding protein p34, a member of the leucine-rich protein family, was found to bind to FGF-1 through its coiled-coil domain (Skjerpen et al. 2002b). This protein is localized in the ER membrane. It was also found that p34, similarly to FIBP and CK2, binds to mitogenic, wild-type FGF-1, but not to the nonmitogenic FGF-1K132E mutant (Skjerpen et al. 2002b; Klingenberg et al. 1998).

Also, FGF-2 interacts with the β-subunit of CK2 and is able to stimulate the kinase (Bonnet et al. 1996). Interestingly, a single mutation (S117A) in the growth factor abolished binding to CK2 and dramatically reduced its mitogenic activity, although it did not abolish the ability of FGF-2 to bind and activate FGFR.

It was reported that the intracellular function of high-molecular-mass isoforms of FGF-2 might be mediated through their interaction with the 55-kD protein FGF-2 interacting factor (FIF), a nuclear polypeptide with putative antiapoptotic properties (Van den et al. 2000). Binding of FIF to FGF-2 was identified by the yeast two-hybrid system. FIF contains a leucine zipper, three hydrophobic heptad repeats, an acidic region, and a bipartite NLS. This protein interacts specifically with FGF-2 but not with FGF-1, FGF-3, or FGF-6. This study also suggests that high-molecular-mass isoforms of FGF-2 act concomitantly with FIF in response to stress (Van den et al. 2000).

Recently, it was reported that the 18-kD isoform of FGF-2 interacts specifically with a cytosolic protein referred to as translokin (Bossard et al. 2003). Translokin colocalizes with the microtubule network and binds to exogenous FGF-2 but not to FGF-1. The protein is involved in mediating nuclear localization of externally added FGF-2. When the expression of translokin was inhibited by siRNA, the nuclear translocation of the growth factor and its mitogenic activity were reduced. The lack of translokin expression had no effect on intracellular FGF-1 trafficking.

Intracellular FGF-3 interacts with NoBP, a protein that contains a nuclear and a nucleolar localization sequence and is accumulated in nucleoli. When overexpressed, NoBP is able to abrogate the cell proliferation inhibitory effect of nuclear FGF-3 (Reimers et al. 2001). It has been shown that the yeast protein Ebp2p, highly related to NoBP, localizes to nucleoli and is required for ribosome biosynthesis and cell growth (Huber et al. 2000). It is not excluded that NoBP can play a similar role in mammalian cells.

For FHFs (FGF-11–14) two intracellular binding partners have been identified. It was shown by a yeast two-hybrid system that FHF1 binds the mitogen-activated protein kinase scaffolding protein islet brain-2 (IB2) (Schoorlemmer and Goldfarb 2001). It has also been proposed that the FHF-IB2 complex is involved in regulating the activity of p38δ MAPK (Schoorlemmer and Goldfarb 2002). The cytoplasmic tails of voltage-gated sodium channels were found to be another intracellular target for

FHFs (Liu et al. 2001). Recently, it was proposed that FHFs can modulate the properties of the cardiac sodium channel Na$_v$1.5 (Liu et al. 2003).

8
Concluding Remarks

An increasing body of evidence indicates that signaling from internalized, activated FGFR is a crucial part of the cellular mechanism of response to FGF stimuli. Formation of a stable FGF-FGFR complex is a prerequisite for this process. Moreover, FGF-1 and -2 are translocated into the cytosol/nucleus of cells, as a result of their internalization. Translocated exogenous FGFs interact with and modulate intracellular targets (Bossard et al. 2003; Skjerpen et al. 2002a), and this is probably an additional mechanism by which FGFs mediate/regulate signaling. On the other hand, endogenous FGF can also participate in regulation of cell proliferation, cell survival, or development of a malignant phenotype. Furthermore, it is not excluded that endogenous as well as exogenous FGFs can control the expression level of each other and FGFRs (Stachowiak et al. 1994). Nuclear/nucleolar localization has also been observed for Let-756, a *C. elegans* FGF (Goldfarb 2001), suggesting that the intracellular function of some FGFs is biologically significant and evolutionarily conserved. In addition to some FGFs, other polypeptide growth factors and cytokines also might act intracellularly. Interferon-γ, IL-1α, prolactin, growth hormone, ciliary neurotrophic factor, lactoferrin, macrophage inhibitory growth factor, and exogenous HIV TAT protein are some examples (Olsnes et al. 2003).

Acknowledgements We wish to thank Prof. Sjur Olsnes, Trine Nilsen, and Jørgen Wesche for critical reading of the manuscript. V.S. is a Post-doctoral Fellow of the Norwegian Cancer Society.

References

Abraham JA, Whang JL, Tumolo A, Mergia A, Friedman J, Gospodarowicz D, Fiddes JC (1986) Human basic fibroblast growth factor: nucleotide sequence and genomic organization. EMBO J 5:2523–2528

Acland P, Dixon M, Peters G, Dickson C (1990) Subcellular fate of the int-2 oncoprotein is determined by choice of initiation codon. Nature 343:662–665

Ahmad SM Baker BS (2002) Sex-specific deployment of FGF signaling in *Drosophila* recruits mesodermal cells into the male genital imaginal disc. Cell 109:651–661

Antoine M, Reimers K, Dickson C, Kiefer P (1997) Fibroblast growth factor 3, a protein with dual subcellular localization, is targeted to the nucleus and nucleolus by the concerted action of two nuclear localization signals and a nucleolar retention signal. J Biol Chem 272:29475–29481

Arese M, Chen Y, Florkiewicz RZ, Gualandris A, Shen B, Rifkin DB (1999) Nuclear activities of basic fibroblast growth factor: Potentiation of low-serum growth mediated by natural or chimeric nuclear localization signals. Mol Biol Cell 10:1429–1444

Arnaud E, Touriol C, Boutonnet C, Gensac MC, Vagner S, Prats H, Prats AC (1999) A new 34-kilodalton isoform of human fibroblast growth factor 2 is cap dependently synthesized by using a non-AUG start codon and behaves as a survival factor. Mol Cell Biol 19:505–514

Baldin V, Roman AM, Bosc-Bierne I, Amalric F, Bouche G (1990) Translocation of bFGF to the nucleus is G1 phase cell cycle specific in bovine aortic endothelial cells. EMBO J 9:1511–1517

Beer HD, Vindevoghel L, Gait MJ, Revest JM, Duan DR, Mason I, Dickson C, Werner S (2000) Fibroblast growth factor (FGF) receptor 1-IIIb is a naturally occurring functional receptor for FGFs that is preferentially expressed in the skin and the brain. J Biol Chem 275:16091–16097

Belleudi F, Ceridono M, Capone A, Serafino A, Marchese C, Picardo M, Frati L, Torrisi MR (2002) The endocytic pathway followed by the keratinocyte growth factor receptor. Histochem Cell Biol 118:1–10

Bikfalvi A, Dupuy E, Inyang AL, Fayein N, Leseche G, Courtois Y, Tobelem G (1989) Binding, internalization, and degradation of basic fibroblast growth factor in human microvascular endothelial cells. Exp Cell Res 181:75–84

Bikfalvi A, Klein S, Pintucci G, Quarto N, Mignatti P, Rifkin DB (1995) Differential modulation of cell phenotype by different molecular weight forms of basic fibroblast growth factor: possible intracellular signaling by the high molecular weight forms. J Cell Biol 129:233–243

Bikfalvi A, Klein S, Pintucci G, Rifkin DB (1997) Biological roles of fibroblast growth factor-2. Endocr Rev 18:26–45

Blaber M, DiSalvo J, Thomas KA (1996) X-ray crystal structure of human acidic fibroblast growth factor. Biochemistry 35:2086–2094

Boilly B, Vercoutter-Edouart AS, Hondermarck H, Nurcombe V, Le B X (2000) FGF signals for cell proliferation and migration through different pathways. Cytokine Growth Factor Rev 11:295–302

Bonnet H, Filhol O, Truchet I, Brethenou P, Cochet C, Amalric F, Bouche G (1996) Fibroblast growth factor-2 binds to the regulatory beta subunit of CK2 and directly stimulates CK2 activity toward nucleolin. J Biol Chem 271:24781–24787

Borland CZ, Schutzman JL, Stern MJ (2001) Fibroblast growth factor signaling in *Caenorhabditis elegans*. Bioessays 23:1120–1130

Bossard C, Laurell H, Van den BL, Meunier S, Zanibellato C, Prats H (2003) Translokin is an intracellular mediator of FGF-2 trafficking. Nat Cell Biol 5:433–439

Bouche G, Gas N, Prats H, Baldin V, Tauber JP, Teissie J, Amalric F (1987) Basic fibroblast growth factor enters the nucleolus and stimulates the transcription of ribosomal genes in ABAE cells undergoing G0-G1 transition. Proc Natl Acad Sci U S A 84:6770–6774

Branda CS Stern MJ (2000) Mechanisms controlling sex myoblast migration in *Caenorhabditis elegans* hermaphrodites. Dev Biol 226:137–151

Brogi E, Winkles JA, Underwood R, Clinton SK, Alberts GF, Libby P (1993) Distinct patterns of expression of fibroblast growth factors and their receptors in human atheroma and nonatherosclerotic arteries. Association of acidic FGF with plaque microvessels and macrophages. J Clin Invest 92:2408–2418

Bugler B, Amalric F, Prats H (1991) Alternative initiation of translation determines cytoplasmic or nuclear localization of basic fibroblast growth factor. Mol Cell Biol 11:573–577

Burdine RD, Chen EB, Kwok SF, Stern MJ (1997) egl-17 encodes an invertebrate fibroblast growth factor family member required specifically for sex myoblast migration in *Caenorhabditis elegans*. Proc Natl Acad Sci U S A 94:2433–2437

Burgess WH, Dionne CA, Kaplow J, Mudd R, Friesel R, Zilberstein A, Schlessinger J, Jaye M (1990) Characterization and cDNA cloning of phospholipase C-gamma, a major substrate for heparin-binding growth factor 1 (acidic fibroblast growth factor)-activated tyrosine kinase. Mol Cell Biol 10:4770–4777

Burgess WH Maciag T (1989) The heparin-binding (fibroblast) growth factor family of proteins. Annu Rev Biochem 58:575–606

Burke D, Wilkes D, Blundell TL, Malcolm S (1998) Fibroblast growth factor receptors: lessons from the genes. Trends Biochem Sci 23:59–62

Burrus LW Olwin BB (1989) Isolation of a receptor for acidic and basic fibroblast growth factor from embryonic chick. J Biol Chem 264:18647–18653

Burrus LW, Zuber ME, Lueddecke BA, Olwin BB (1992) Identification of a cysteine-rich receptor for fibroblast growth factors. Mol Cell Biol 12:5600–5609

Cao Y, Ekstrom M, Pettersson RF (1993) Characterization of the nuclear translocation of acidic fibroblast growth factor. J Cell Sci 104 (Pt 1):77–87

Cavallaro U, Niedermeyer J, Fuxa M, Christofori G (2001) N-CAM modulates tumour-cell adhesion to matrix by inducing FGF-receptor signalling. Nat Cell Biol 3:650–657

Celli G, LaRochelle WJ, Mackem S, Sharp R, Merlino G (1998) Soluble dominant-negative receptor uncovers essential roles for fibroblast growth factors in multiorgan induction and patterning. EMBO J 17:1642–1655

Ciruna B Rossant J (2001) FGF signaling regulates mesoderm cell fate specification and morphogenetic movement at the primitive streak. Dev Cell 1:37–49

Citores L, Khnykin D, Sorensen V, Wesche J, Klingenberg O, Wiedlocha A, Olsnes S (2001) Modulation of intracellular transport of acidic fibroblast growth factor by mutations in the cytoplasmic receptor domain. J Cell Sci 114:1677–1689

Citores L, Wesche J, Kolpakova E, Olsnes S (1999) Uptake and intracellular transport of acidic fibroblast growth factor: evidence for free and cytoskeleton-anchored fibroblast growth factor receptors. Mol Biol Cell 10:3835–3848

Clarke S (1992) Protein isoprenylation and methylation at carboxyl-terminal cysteine residues. Annu Rev Biochem 61:355–386

Cleves AE (1997) Protein transports: the nonclassical ins and outs. Curr Biol 7:R318-R320

Copeland RA, Ji H, Halfpenny AJ, Williams RW, Thompson KC, Herber WK, Thomas KA, Bruner MW, Ryan JA, Marquis-Omer D (1991) The structure of human acidic fibroblast growth factor and its interaction with heparin. Arch Biochem Biophys 289:53–61

Coulier F, Pontarotti P, Roubin R, Hartung H, Goldfarb M, Birnbaum D (1997) Of worms and men: an evolutionary perspective on the fibroblast growth factor (FGF) and FGF receptor families. J Mol Evol 44:43–56

Cross MJ, Lu L, Magnusson P, Nyqvist D, Holmqvist K, Welsh M, Claesson-Welsh L (2002) The Shb adaptor protein binds to tyrosine 766 in the FGFR-1 and regulates the Ras/MEK/MAPK pathway via FRS2 phosphorylation in endothelial cells. Mol Biol Cell 13:2881–2893

Cuevas P, Gonzalez AM, Carceller F, Baird A (1991) Vascular response to basic fibroblast growth factor when infused onto the normal adventitia or into the injured media of the rat carotid artery. Circ Res 69:360–369

Dahl JP, Binda A, Canfield VA, Levenson R (2000) Participation of Na,K-ATPase in FGF-2 secretion: rescue of ouabain-inhibitable FGF-2 secretion by ouabain-resistant Na,K-ATPase alpha subunits. Biochemistry 39:14877–14883

De Moerlooze L Dickson C (1997) Skeletal disorders associated with fibroblast growth factor receptor mutations. Curr Opin Genet Dev 7:378–385

Delehedde M, Seve M, Sergeant N, Wartelle I, Lyon M, Rudland PS, Fernig DG (2000) Fibroblast growth factor-2 stimulation of p42/44MAPK phosphorylation and IkappaB degradation is regulated by heparan sulfate/heparin in rat mammary fibroblasts. J Biol Chem 275:33905–33910

Eriksson AE, Cousens LS, Weaver LH, Matthews BW (1991) Three-dimensional structure of human basic fibroblast growth factor. Proc Natl Acad Sci U S A 88:3441–3445

Ezzat S, Zheng L, Zhu XF, Wu GE, Asa SL (2002) Targeted expression of a human pituitary tumor-derived isoform of FGF receptor-4 recapitulates pituitary tumorigenesis. J Clin Invest 109:69–78

Fannon M Nugent MA (1996) Basic fibroblast growth factor binds its receptors, is internalized, and stimulates DNA synthesis in Balb/c3T3 cells in the absence of heparan sulfate. J Biol Chem 271:17949–17956

Florkiewicz RZ, Anchin J, Baird A (1998) The inhibition of fibroblast growth factor-2 export by cardenolides implies a novel function for the catalytic subunit of Na$^+$,K$^+$-ATPase. J Biol Chem 273:544–551

Florkiewicz RZ, Majack RA, Buechler RD, Florkiewicz E (1995) Quantitative export of FGF-2 occurs through an alternative, energy-dependent, non-ER/Golgi pathway. J Cell Physiol 162:388–399

Florkiewicz RZ Sommer A (1989) Human basic fibroblast growth factor gene encodes four polypeptides: three initiate translation from non-AUG codons. Proc Natl Acad Sci U S A 86:3978–3981

Friedman S, Zhan X, Maciag T (1994) Mutagenesis of the nuclear localization sequence in EGF-1 alters protein stability but not mitogenic activity. Biochem Biophys Res Commun 198:1203–1208

Friesel R Maciag T (1988) Internalization and degradation of heparin binding growth factor-I by endothelial cells. Biochem Biophys Res Commun 151:957–964

Friesel RE Maciag T (1995) Molecular mechanisms of angiogenesis: fibroblast growth factor signal transduction. FASEB J 9:919–925

Galzie Z, Kinsella AR, Smith JA (1997) Fibroblast growth factors and their receptors. Biochem Cell Biol 75:669–685

Gao G Goldfarb M (1995) Heparin can activate a receptor tyrosine kinase. EMBO J 14:2183–2190

Gleizes PE, Noaillac-Depeyre J, Amalric F, Gas N (1995) Basic fibroblast growth factor (FGF-2) internalization through the heparan sulfate proteoglycans-mediated pathway: an ultrastructural approach. Eur J Cell Biol 66:47–59

Gleizes PE, Noaillac-Depeyre J, Dupont MA, Gas N (1996) Basic fibroblast growth factor (FGF-2) is addressed to caveolae after binding to the plasma membrane of BHK cells. Eur J Cell Biol 71:144–153

Goldfarb M (1996) Functions of fibroblast growth factors in vertebrate development. Cytokine Growth Factor Rev 7:311–325

Goldfarb M (2001) Signaling by fibroblast growth factors: the inside story. Sci STKE 2001:E37

Goldstrohm AC, Greenleaf AL, Garcia-Blanco MA (2001) Co-transcriptional splicing of pre-messenger RNAs: considerations for the mechanism of alternative splicing. Gene 277:31–47

Gonatas JO, Mourelatos Z, Stieber A, Lane WS, Brosius J, Gonatas NK (1995) MG-160, a membrane sialoglycoprotein of the medial cisternae of the rat Golgi apparatus, binds basic fibroblast growth factor and exhibits a high level of sequence identity to a chicken fibroblast growth factor receptor. J Cell Sci 108 (Pt 2):457–467

Grieb TA Burgess WH (2000) The mitogenic activity of fibroblast growth factor-1 correlates with its internalization and limited proteolytic processing. J Cell Physiol 184:171–182

Guillonneau X, Regnier-Ricard F, Laplace O, Jonet L, Bryckaert M, Courtois Y, Mascarelli F (1998) Fibroblast growth factor (FGF) soluble receptor 1 acts as a natural inhibitor of FGF2 neurotrophic activity during retinal degeneration. Mol Biol Cell 9:2785–2802

Gupta S, Aggarwal S, Nakamura S (1998) A possible role of multidrug resistance-associated protein (MRP) in basic fibroblast growth factor secretion by AIDS-associated Kaposi's sarcoma cells: a survival molecule? J Clin Immunol 18:256–263

Halaban R (1996) Growth factors and melanomas. Semin Oncol 23:673–681

Hanafusa H, Torii S, Yasunaga T, Nishida E (2002) Sprouty1 and Sprouty2 provide a control mechanism for the Ras/MAPK signalling pathway. Nat Cell Biol 4:850–858

Hanneken A, Maher PA, Baird A (1995) High affinity immunoreactive FGF receptors in the extracellular matrix of vascular endothelial cells–implications for the modulation of FGF-2. J Cell Biol 128:1221–1228

Hanneken A, Ying W, Ling N, Baird A (1994) Identification of soluble forms of the fibroblast growth factor receptor in blood. Proc Natl Acad Sci U S A 91:9170–9174

Heldin CH Ostman A (1996) Ligand-induced dimerization of growth factor receptors: variations on the theme. Cytokine Growth Factor Rev 7:3–10

Horowitz A, Tkachenko E, Simons M (2002) Fibroblast growth factor-specific modulation of cellular response by syndecan-4. J Cell Biol 157:715–725

Huber MD, Dworet JH, Shire K, Frappier L, McAlear MA (2000) The budding yeast homolog of the human EBNA1-binding protein 2 (Ebp2p) is an essential nucleolar protein required for pre-rRNA processing. J Biol Chem 275:28764–28773

Hughes SE (1996) Localisation and differential expression of the fibroblast growth factor receptor (FGFR) multigene family in normal and atherosclerotic human arteries. Cardiovasc Res 32:557–569

Imamura T, Engleka K, Zhan X, Tokita Y, Forough R, Roeder D, Jackson A, Maier JA, Hla T, Maciag T (1990) Recovery of mitogenic activity of a growth factor mutant with a nuclear translocation sequence. Science 249:1567–1570

Imamura T, Oka S, Tanahashi T, Okita Y (1994) Cell cycle-dependent nuclear localization of exogenously added fibroblast growth factor-1 in BALB/c 3T3 and human vascular endothelial cells. Exp Cell Res 215:363–372

Imamura T, Tokita Y, Mitsui Y (1992) Identification of a heparin-binding growth factor-1 nuclear translocation sequence by deletion mutation analysis. J Biol Chem 267:5676–5679

Jackson A, Friedman S, Zhan X, Engleka KA, Forough R, Maciag T (1992) Heat shock induces the release of fibroblast growth factor 1 from NIH 3T3 cells. Proc Natl Acad Sci U S A 89:10691–10695

Jackson A, Tarantini F, Gamble S, Friedman S, Maciag T (1995) The release of fibroblast growth factor-1 from NIH 3T3 cells in response to temperature involves the function of cysteine residues. J Biol Chem 270:33–36

Jang JH (2002) Identification and characterization of soluble isoform of fibroblast growth factor receptor 3 in human SaOS-2 osteosarcoma cells. Biochem Biophys Res Commun 292:378–382

Jans DA Hassan G (1998) Nuclear targeting by growth factors, cytokines, and their receptors: a role in signaling? Bioessays 20:400–411

Jaye M, Howk R, Burgess W, Ricca GA, Chiu IM, Ravera MW, O'Brien SJ, Modi WS, Maciag T, Drohan WN (1986) Human endothelial cell growth factor: cloning, nucleotide sequence, and chromosome localization. Science 233:541–545

Johnson DE, Lee PL, Lu J, Williams LT (1990) Diverse forms of a receptor for acidic and basic fibroblast growth factors. Mol Cell Biol 10:4728–4736

Johnson DE, Lu J, Chen H, Werner S, Williams LT (1991) The human fibroblast growth factor receptor genes: a common structural arrangement underlies the mechanisms for generating receptor forms that differ in their third immunoglobulin domain. Mol Cell Biol 11:4627–4634

Johnson DE Williams LT (1993) Structural and functional diversity in the FGF receptor multigene family. Adv Cancer Res 60:1–41

Johnston CL, Cox HC, Gomm JJ, Coombes RC (1995) Fibroblast growth factor receptors (FGFRs) localize in different cellular compartments. A splice variant of FGFR-3 localizes to the nucleus. J Biol Chem 270:30643–30650

Joy A, Moffett J, Neary K, Mordechai E, Stachowiak EK, Coons S, Rankin-Shapiro J, Florkiewicz RZ, Stachowiak MK (1997) Nuclear accumulation of FGF-2 is associated with proliferation of human astrocytes and glioma cells. Oncogene 14:171–183

Kan M, Wang F, Xu J, Crabb JW, Hou J, McKeehan WL (1993) An essential heparin-binding domain in the fibroblast growth factor receptor kinase. Science 259:1918–1921

Kiefer P, Acland P, Pappin D, Peters G, Dickson C (1994) Competition between nuclear localization and secretory signals determines the subcellular fate of a single CUG-initiated form of FGF3. EMBO J 13:4126–4136

Kiefer P Dickson C (1995) Nucleolar association of fibroblast growth factor 3 via specific sequence motifs has inhibitory effects on cell growth. Mol Cell Biol 15:4364–4374

Klagsbrun M Baird A (1991) A dual receptor system is required for basic fibroblast growth factor activity. Cell 67:229–231

Klambt C, Glazer L, Shilo BZ (1992) breathless, a Drosophila FGF receptor homolog, is essential for migration of tracheal and specific midline glial cells. Genes Dev 6:1668–1678

Klingenberg O, Widlocha A, Rapak A, Munoz R, Falnes P, Olsnes S (1998) Inability of the acidic fibroblast growth factor mutant K132E to stimulate DNA synthesis after translocation into cells. J Biol Chem 273:11164–11172

Klingenberg O, Wiedlocha A, Rapak A, Khnykin D, Citores L, Olsnes S (2000a) Requirement for C-terminal end of fibroblast growth factor receptor 4 in translocation of acidic fibroblast growth factor to cytosol and nucleus. J Cell Sci 113 (Pt 10):1827–1838

Klingenberg O, Wiedocha A, Citores L, Olsnes S (2000b) Requirement of phosphatidylinositol 3-kinase activity for translocation of exogenous aFGF to the cytosol and nucleus. J Biol Chem 275:11972–11980

Klint P Claesson-Welsh L (1999) Signal transduction by fibroblast growth factor receptors. Front Biosci 4:D165–D177

Klint P, Kanda S, Claesson-Welsh L (1995) Shc and a novel 89-kDa component couple to the Grb2-Sos complex in fibroblast growth factor-2-stimulated cells. J Biol Chem 270:23337–23344

Kohl R, Antoine M, Olwin BB, Dickson C, Kiefer P (2000) Cysteine-rich fibroblast growth factor receptor alters secretion and intracellular routing of fibroblast growth factor 3. J Biol Chem 275:15741–15748

Kolpakova E, Wiedlocha A, Stenmark H, Klingenberg O, Falnes PO, Olsnes S (1998) Cloning of an intracellular protein that binds selectively to mitogenic acidic fibroblast growth factor. Biochem J 336 (Pt 1):213–222

Kouhara H, Hadari YR, Spivak-Kroizman T, Schilling J, Bar-Sagi D, Lax I, Schlessinger J (1997) A lipid-anchored Grb2-binding protein that links FGF-receptor activation to the Ras/MAPK signaling pathway. Cell 89:693–702

Kovalenko D, Yang X, Nadeau RJ, Harkins LK, Friesel R (2003) Sef inhibits fibroblast growth factor signaling by inhibiting FGFR1 tyrosine phosphorylation and subsequent ERK activation. J Biol Chem 278:14087–14091

Lander ES, Linton LM, Birren B, Nusbaum C, Zody MC, Baldwin J, Devon K, Dewar K, Doyle M, FitzHugh W, Funke R, Gage D, Harris K, Heaford A, Howland J, Kann L, Lehoczky J, LeVine R, McEwan P, McKernan K, Meldrim J, Mesirov JP, Miranda C, Morris W, Naylor J, Raymond C, Rosetti M, Santos R, Sheridan A, Sougnez C, Stange-Thomann N, Stojanovic N, Subramanian A, Wyman D, Rogers J, Sulston J, Ainscough R, Beck S, Bentley D, Burton J, Clee C, Carter N, Coulson A, Deadman R, Deloukas P, Dunham A, Dunham I, Durbin R, French L, Grafham D, Gregory S, Hubbard T, Humphray S, Hunt A, Jones M, Lloyd C, McMurray A, Matthews L, Mercer S, Milne S, Mullikin JC, Mungall A, Plumb R, Ross M, Shownkeen R, Sims

S, Waterston RH, Wilson RK, Hillier LW, McPherson JD, Marra MA, Mardis ER, Fulton LA, Chinwalla AT, Pepin KH, Gish WR, Chissoe SL, Wendl MC, Delehaunty KD, Miner TL, Delehaunty A, Kramer JB, Cook LL, Fulton RS, Johnson DL, Minx PJ, Clifton SW, Hawkins T, Branscomb E, Predki P, Richardson P, Wenning S, Slezak T, Doggett N, Cheng JF, Olsen A, Lucas S, Elkin C, Uberbacher E, Frazier M, Gibbs RA, Muzny DM, Scherer SE, Bouck JB, Sodergren EJ, Worley KC, Rives CM, Gorrell JH, Metzker ML, Naylor SL, Kucherlapati RS, Nelson DL, Weinstock GM, Sakaki Y, Fujiyama A, Hattori M, Yada T, Toyoda A, Itoh T, Kawagoe C, Watanabe H, Totoki Y, Taylor T, Weissenbach J, Heilig R, Saurin W, Artiguenave F, Brottier P, Bruls T, Pelletier E, Robert C, Wincker P, Smith DR, Doucette-Stamm L, Rubenfield M, Weinstock K, Lee HM, Dubois J, Rosenthal A, Platzer M, Nyakatura G, Taudien S, Rump A, Yang H, Yu J, Wang J, Huang G, Gu J, Hood L, Rowen L, Madan A, Qin S, Davis RW, Federspiel NA, Abola AP, Proctor MJ, Myers RM, Schmutz J, Dickson M, Grimwood J, Cox DR, Olson MV, Kaul R, Raymond C, Shimizu N, Kawasaki K, Minoshima S, Evans GA, Athanasiou M, Schultz R, Roe BA, Chen F, Pan H, Ramser J, Lehrach H, Reinhardt R, McCombie WR, de la BM, Dedhia N, Blocker H, Hornischer K, Nordsiek G, Agarwala R, Aravind L, Bailey JA, Bateman A, Batzoglou S, Birney E, Bork P, Brown DG, Burge CB, Cerutti L, Chen HC, Church D, Clamp M, Copley RR, Doerks T, Eddy SR, Eichler EE, Furey TS, Galagan J, Gilbert JG, Harmon C, Hayashizaki Y, Haussler D, Hermjakob H, Hokamp K, Jang W, Johnson LS, Jones TA, Kasif S, Kaspryzk A, Kennedy S, Kent WJ, Kitts P, Koonin EV, Korf I, Kulp D, Lancet D, Lowe TM, McLysaght A, Mikkelsen T, Moran JV, Mulder N, Pollara VJ, Ponting CP, Schuler G, Schultz J, Slater G, Smit AF, Stupka E, Szustakowski J, Thierry-Mieg D, Thierry-Mieg J, Wagner L, Wallis J, Wheeler R, Williams A, Wolf YI, Wolfe KH, Yang SP, Yeh RF, Collins F, Guyer MS, Peterson J, Felsenfeld A, Wetterstrand KA, Patrinos A, Morgan MJ, Szustakowki J, de Jong P, Catanese JJ, Osoegawa K, Shizuya H, Choi S (2001) Initial sequencing and analysis of the human genome. Nature 409:860–921

Landgren E, Blume-Jensen P, Courtneidge SA, Claesson-Welsh L (1995) Fibroblast growth factor receptor-1 regulation of Src family kinases. Oncogene 10:2027–2035

Larsson H, Klint P, Landgren E, Claesson-Welsh L (1999) Fibroblast growth factor receptor-1-mediated endothelial cell proliferation is dependent on the Src homology (SH) 2/SH3 domain-containing adaptor protein Crk. J Biol Chem 274:25726–25734

LaVallee TM, Prudovsky IA, McMahon GA, Hu X, Maciag T (1998) Activation of the MAP kinase pathway by FGF-1 correlates with cell proliferation induction while activation of the Src pathway correlates with migration. J Cell Biol 141:1647–1658

Lax I, Wong A, Lamothe B, Lee A, Frost A, Hawes J, Schlessinger J (2002) The docking protein FRS2alpha controls a MAP kinase-mediated negative feedback mechanism for signaling by FGF receptors. Mol Cell 10:709–719

Li Y, Basilico C, Mansukhani A (1994) Cell transformation by fibroblast growth factors can be suppressed by truncated fibroblast growth factor receptors. Mol Cell Biol 14:7660–7669

Liau G, Winkles JA, Cannon MS, Kuo L, Chilian WM (1993) Dietary-induced atherosclerotic lesions have increased levels of acidic FGF mRNA and altered cytoskeletal and extracellular matrix mRNA expression. J Vasc Res 30:327–332

Lim YP, Low BC, Lim J, Wong ES, Guy GR (1999) Association of atypical protein kinase C isotypes with the docker protein FRS2 in fibroblast growth factor signaling. J Biol Chem 274:19025–19034

Lin X, Buff EM, Perrimon N, Michelson AM (1999) Heparan sulfate proteoglycans are essential for FGF receptor signaling during *Drosophila* embryonic development. Development 126:3715–3723

Liu CJ, Dib-Hajj SD, Black JA, Greenwood J, Lian Z, Waxman SG (2001) Direct interaction with contactin targets voltage-gated sodium channel Na(v)1.9/NaN to the cell membrane. J Biol Chem 276:46553–46561

Liu CJ, Dib-Hajj SD, Renganathan M, Cummins TR, Waxman SG (2003) Modulation of the cardiac sodium channel Nav1.5 by fibroblast growth factor homologous factor 1B. J Biol Chem 278:1029–1036

Liu J, Huang C, Zhan X (1999) Src is required for cell migration and shape changes induced by fibroblast growth factor 1. Oncogene 18:6700–6706

Lundin L, Larsson H, Kreuger J, Kanda S, Lindahl U, Salmivirta M, Claesson-Welsh L (2000) Selectively desulfated heparin inhibits fibroblast growth factor-induced mitogenicity and angiogenesis. J Biol Chem 275:24653–24660

Lundin L, Ronnstrand L, Cross M, Hellberg C, Lindahl U, Claesson-Welsh L (2003) Differential tyrosine phosphorylation of fibroblast growth factor (FGF) receptor-1 and receptor proximal signal transduction in response to FGF-2 and heparin. Exp Cell Res 287:190–198

Mach H, Middaugh CR (1995) Interaction of partially structured states of acidic fibroblast growth factor with phospholipid membranes. Biochemistry 34:9913–9920

Maciag T Friesel RE (1995) Molecular mechanisms of fibroblast growth factor-1 traffic, signaling and release. Thromb Haemost 74:411–414

Maher PA (1996) Nuclear translocation of fibroblast growth factor (FGF) receptors in response to FGF-2. J Cell Biol 134:529–536

Malecki J, Wiedlocha A, Wesche J, Olsnes S (2002) Vesicle transmembrane potential is required for translocation to the cytosol of externally added FGF-1. EMBO J 21:4480–4490

Marchese C, Mancini P, Belleudi F, Felici A, Gradini R, Sansolini T, Frati L, Torrisi MR (1998) Receptor-mediated endocytosis of keratinocyte growth factor. J Cell Sci 111 (Pt 23):3517–3527

Martin GR (1998) The roles of FGFs in the early development of vertebrate limbs. Genes Dev 12:1571–1586

Mason I (2003) Fibroblast growth factors. Curr Biol 13:R346

McNeil PL Steinhardt RA (1997) Loss, restoration, and maintenance of plasma membrane integrity. J Cell Biol 137:1–4

Mignatti P, Morimoto T, Rifkin DB (1992) Basic fibroblast growth factor, a protein devoid of secretory signal sequence, is released by cells via a pathway independent of the endoplasmic reticulum-Golgi complex. J Cell Physiol 151:81–93

Mignatti P Rifkin DB (1991) Release of basic fibroblast growth factor, an angiogenic factor devoid of secretory signal sequence: a trivial phenomenon or a novel secretion mechanism? J Cell Biochem 47:201–207

Miyake A, Konishi M, Martin FH, Hernday NA, Ozaki K, Yamamoto S, Mikami T, Arakawa T, Itoh N (1998) Structure and expression of a novel member, FGF-16, on the fibroblast growth factor family. Biochem Biophys Res Commun 243:148–152

Miyamoto M, Naruo K, Seko C, Matsumoto S, Kondo T, Kurokawa T (1993) Molecular cloning of a novel cytokine cDNA encoding the ninth member of the fibroblast growth factor family, which has a unique secretion property. Mol Cell Biol 13:4251–4259

Mizukoshi E, Suzuki M, Loupatov A, Uruno T, Hayashi H, Misono T, Kaul SC, Wadhwa R, Imamura T (1999) Fibroblast growth factor-1 interacts with the glucose-regulated protein GRP75/mortalin. Biochem J 343 Pt 2:461–466

Moenner M, Gannoun-Zaki L, Badet J, Barritault D (1989) Internalization and limited processing of basic fibroblast growth factor on Chinese hamster lung fibroblasts. Growth Factors 1:115–123

Mohammadi M, Honegger AM, Rotin D, Fischer R, Bellot F, Li W, Dionne CA, Jaye M, Rubinstein M, Schlessinger J (1991) A tyrosine-phosphorylated carboxy-terminal peptide of the fibroblast growth factor receptor (Flg) is a binding site for the SH2 domain of phospholipase C-gamma 1. Mol Cell Biol 11:5068–5078

Monsonego-Ornan E, Adar R, Rom E, Yayon A (2002) FGF receptors ubiquitylation: dependence on tyrosine kinase activity and role in downregulation. FEBS Lett 528:83–89

Mori S, Claesson-Welsh L, Okuyama Y, Saito Y (1995) Ligand-induced polyubiquitination of receptor tyrosine kinases. Biochem Biophys Res Commun 213:32–39

Moscatelli D (1988) Metabolism of receptor-bound and matrix-bound basic fibroblast growth factor by bovine capillary endothelial cells. J Cell Biol 107:753–759

Moscatelli D Devesly P (1990) Turnover of functional basic fibroblast growth factor receptors on the surface of BHK and NIH 3T3 cells. Growth Factors 3:25–33

Mourelatos Z, Gonatas JO, Cinato E, Gonatas NK (1996) Cloning and sequence analysis of the human MG160, a fibroblast growth factor and E-selectin binding membrane sialoglycoprotein of the Golgi apparatus. DNA Cell Biol 15:1121–1128

Mouta CC, LaVallee TM, Tarantini F, Jackson A, Lathrop JT, Hampton B, Burgess WH, Maciag T (1998) S100A13 is involved in the regulation of fibroblast growth factor-1 and p40 synaptotagmin-1 release in vitro. J Biol Chem 273:22224–22231

Munoz-Sanjuan I, Simandl BK, Fallon JF, Nathans J (1999) Expression of chicken fibroblast growth factor homologous factor (FHF)-1 and of differentially spliced isoforms of FHF-2 during development and involvement of FHF-2 in chicken limb development. Development 126:409–421

Munoz-Sanjuan I, Smallwood PM, Nathans J (2000) Isoform diversity among fibroblast growth factor homologous factors is generated by alternative promoter usage and differential splicing. J Biol Chem 275:2589–2597

Munoz R, Klingenberg O, Wiedlocha A, Rapak A, Falnes PO, Olsnes S (1997) Effect of mutation of cytoplasmic receptor domain and of genistein on transport of acidic fibroblast growth factor into cells. Oncogene 15:525–536

Myers JM, Martins GG, Ostrowski J, Stachowiak MK (2003) Nuclear trafficking of FGFR1: A role for the transmembrane domain. J Cell Biochem 88:1273–1291

Nagendra HG, Harrington AE, Harmer NJ, Pellegrini L, Blundell TL, Burke DF (2001) Sequence analyses and comparative modeling of fly and worm fibroblast growth factor receptors indicate that the determinants for FGF and heparin binding are retained in evolution. FEBS Lett 501:51–58

Nakanishi Y, Kihara K, Mizuno K, Masamune Y, Yoshitake Y, Nishikawa K (1992) Direct effect of basic fibroblast growth factor on gene transcription in a cell-free system. Proc Natl Acad Sci U S A 89:5216–5220

Naski MC Ornitz DM (1998) FGF signaling in skeletal development. Front Biosci 3:D781-D794

Ohmachi S, Watanabe Y, Mikami T, Kusu N, Ibi T, Akaike A, Itoh N (2000) FGF-20, a novel neurotrophic factor, preferentially expressed in the substantia nigra pars compacta of rat brain. Biochem Biophys Res Commun 277:355–360

Okada-Ban M, Moens G, Thiery JP, Jouanneau J (1999) Nuclear 24 kD fibroblast growth factor (FGF)-2 confers metastatic properties on rat bladder carcinoma cells. Oncogene 18:6719–6724

Olsen SK, Garbi M, Zampieri N, Eliseenkova AV, Ornitz DM, Goldfarb M, Mohammadi M (2003) Fibroblast growth factor (FGF) homologous factors share structural but not functional homology with FGFs. J Biol Chem 278:34226–34236

Olsnes S, Klingenberg O, Wiedlocha A (2003) Transport of exogenous growth factors and cytokines to the cytosol and to the nucleus. Physiol Rev 83:163–182

Ong SH, Guy GR, Hadari YR, Laks S, Gotoh N, Schlessinger J, Lax I (2000) FRS2 proteins recruit intracellular signaling pathways by binding to diverse targets on fibroblast growth factor and nerve growth factor receptors. Mol Cell Biol 20:979–989

Ong SH, Hadari YR, Gotoh N, Guy GR, Schlessinger J, Lax I (2001) Stimulation of phosphatidylinositol 3-kinase by fibroblast growth factor receptors is mediated by coordinated recruitment of multiple docking proteins. Proc Natl Acad Sci U S A 98:6074–6079

Ornitz DM (2000) FGFs, heparan sulfate and FGFRs: complex interactions essential for development. Bioessays 22:108–112

Ornitz DM Itoh N (2001) Fibroblast growth factors. Genome Biol 2:REVIEWS3005

Ornitz DM Marie PJ (2002) FGF signaling pathways in endochondral and intramembranous bone development and human genetic disease. Genes Dev 16:1446–1465

Ornitz DM, Yayon A, Flanagan JG, Svahn CM, Levi E, Leder P (1992) Heparin is required for cell-free binding of basic fibroblast growth factor to a soluble receptor and for mitogenesis in whole cells. Mol Cell Biol 12:240–247

Orr-Urtreger A, Bedford MT, Burakova T, Arman E, Zimmer Y, Yayon A, Givol D, Lonai P (1993) Developmental localization of the splicing alternatives of fibroblast growth factor receptor-2 (FGFR2). Dev Biol 158:475–486

Ozawa K, Suzuki S, Asada M, Tomooka Y, Li AJ, Yoneda A, Komi A, Imamura T (1998) An alternatively spliced fibroblast growth factor (FGF)-5 mRNA is abundant in brain and translates into a partial agonist/antagonist for FGF-5 neurotrophic activity. J Biol Chem 273:29262–29271

Patry V, Bugler B, Maret A, Potier M, Prats H (1997) Endogenous basic fibroblast growth factor isoforms involved in different intracellular protein complexes. Biochem J 326 (Pt 1):259–264

Pellegrini L, Burke DF, von Delft F, Mulloy B, Blundell TL (2000) Crystal structure of fibroblast growth factor receptor ectodomain bound to ligand and heparin. Nature 407:1029–1034

Pineda-Lucena A, Nunez DC, I, Lozano RM, Munoz-Willery I, Zazo M, Gimenez-Gallego G (1994) Effect of low pH and heparin on the structure of acidic fibroblast growth factor. Eur J Biochem 222:425–431

Piotrowicz RS, Martin JL, Dillman WH, Levin EG (1997) The 27-kDa heat shock protein facilitates basic fibroblast growth factor release from endothelial cells. J Biol Chem 272:7042–7047

Plopper GE, McNamee HP, Dike LE, Bojanowski K, Ingber DE (1995) Convergence of integrin and growth factor receptor signaling pathways within the focal adhesion complex. Mol Biol Cell 6:1349–1365

Plotnikov AN, Hubbard SR, Schlessinger J, Mohammadi M (2000) Crystal structures of two FGF-FGFR complexes reveal the determinants of ligand-receptor specificity. Cell 101:413–424

Plotnikov AN, Schlessinger J, Hubbard SR, Mohammadi M (1999) Structural basis for FGF receptor dimerization and activation. Cell 98:641–650

Powell PP Klagsbrun M (1991) Three forms of rat basic fibroblast growth factor are made from a single mRNA and localize to the nucleus. J Cell Physiol 148:202–210

Powers CJ, McLeskey SW, Wellstein A (2000) Fibroblast growth factors, their receptors and signaling. Endocr Relat Cancer 7:165–197

Prats H, Kaghad M, Prats AC, Klagsbrun M, Lelias JM, Liauzun P, Chalon P, Tauber JP, Amalric F, Smith JA (1989) High molecular mass forms of basic fibroblast growth factor are initiated by alternative CUG codons. Proc Natl Acad Sci U S A 86:1836–1840

Prudovsky I, Bagala C, Tarantini F, Mandinova A, Soldi R, Bellum S, Maciag T (2002) The intracellular translocation of the components of the fibroblast growth factor 1 release complex precedes their assembly prior to export. J Cell Biol 158:201–208

Pursiheimo JP, Jalkanen M, Tasken K, Jaakkola P (2000) Involvement of protein kinase A in fibroblast growth factor-2-activated transcription. Proc Natl Acad Sci U S A 97:168–173

Pursiheimo JP, Kieksi A, Jalkanen M, Salmivirta M (2002a) Protein kinase A balances the growth factor-induced Ras/ERK signaling. FEBS Lett 521:157–164

Pursiheimo JP, Saari J, Jalkanen M, Salmivirta M (2002b) Cooperation of protein kinase A and Ras/ERK signaling pathways is required for AP-1-mediated activation of fibroblast growth factor-inducible response element (FiRE). J Biol Chem 277:25344–25355

Rapraeger AC, Krufka A, Olwin BB (1991) Requirement of heparan sulfate for bFGF-mediated fibroblast growth and myoblast differentiation. Science 252:1705–1708

Reilly JF Maher PA (2001) Importin beta-mediated nuclear import of fibroblast growth factor receptor: Role in cell proliferation. J Cell Biol 152:1307–1312

Reimers K, Antoine M, Zapatka M, Blecken V, Dickson C, Kiefer P (2001) NoBP, a nuclear fibroblast growth factor 3 binding protein, is cell cycle regulated and promotes cell growth. Mol Cell Biol 21:4996–5007

Rieck P, Hartmann C, Jacob C, Pouliquen Y, Courtois Y (1992) Human recombinant bFGF stimulates corneal endothelial wound healing in rabbits. Curr Eye Res 11:1161–1172

Riese J, Zeller R, Dono R (1995) Nucleo-cytoplasmic translocation and secretion of fibroblast growth factor-2 during avian gastrulation. Mech Dev 49:13–22

Roghani M Moscatelli D (1992) Basic fibroblast growth factor is internalized through both receptor-mediated and heparan sulfate-mediated mechanisms. J Biol Chem 267:22156–22162

Ruoslahti E Yamaguchi Y (1991) Proteoglycans as modulators of growth factor activities. Cell 64:867–869

Sakaguchi K, Lorenzi MV, Bottaro DP, Miki T (1999) The acidic domain and first immunoglobulin-like loop of fibroblast growth factor receptor 2 modulate downstream signaling through glycosaminoglycan modification. Mol Cell Biol 19:6754–6764

Sano H, Forough R, Maier JA, Case JP, Jackson A, Engleka K, Maciag T, Wilder RL (1990) Detection of high levels of heparin binding growth factor-1 (acidic fibroblast growth factor) in inflammatory arthritic joints. J Cell Biol 110:1417–1426

Schlessinger J (2000) Cell signaling by receptor tyrosine kinases. Cell 103:211–225

Schlessinger J (2003) Signal transduction. Autoinhibition control. Science 300:750–752

Schlessinger J, Plotnikov AN, Ibrahimi OA, Eliseenkova AV, Yeh BK, Yayon A, Linhardt RJ, Mohammadi M (2000) Crystal structure of a ternary FGF-FGFR-heparin complex reveals a dual role for heparin in FGFR binding and dimerization. Mol Cell 6:743–750

Schoorlemmer J Goldfarb M (2001) Fibroblast growth factor homologous factors are intracellular signaling proteins. Curr Biol 11:793–797

Schoorlemmer J Goldfarb M (2002) Fibroblast growth factor homologous factors and the islet brain-2 scaffold protein regulate activation of a stress-activated protein kinase. J Biol Chem 277:49111–49119

Sherman L, Stocker KM, Morrison R, Ciment G (1993) Basic fibroblast growth factor (bFGF) acts intracellularly to cause the transdifferentiation of avian neural crest-derived Schwann cell precursors into melanocytes. Development 118:1313–1326

Shiang R, Thompson LM, Zhu YZ, Church DM, Fielder TJ, Bocian M, Winokur ST, Wasmuth JJ (1994) Mutations in the transmembrane domain of FGFR3 cause the most common genetic form of dwarfism, achondroplasia. Cell 78:335–342

Shin JT, Opalenik SR, Wehby JN, Mahesh VK, Jackson A, Tarantini F, Maciag T, Thompson JA (1996) Serum-starvation induces the extracellular appearance of FGF-1. Biochim Biophys Acta 1312:27–38

Skjerpen CS, Nilsen T, Wesche J, Olsnes S (2002a) Binding of FGF-1 variants to protein kinase CK2 correlates with mitogenicity. EMBO J 21:4058–4069

Skjerpen CS, Wesche J, Olsnes S (2002b) Identification of ribosome-binding protein p34 as an intracellular protein that binds acidic fibroblast growth factor. J Biol Chem 277:23864–23871

Sleeman M, Fraser J, McDonald M, Yuan S, White D, Grandison P, Kumble K, Watson JD, Murison JG (2001) Identification of a new fibroblast growth factor receptor, FGFR5. Gene 271:171–182

Smallwood PM, Munoz-Sanjuan I, Tong P, Macke JP, Hendry SH, Gilbert DJ, Copeland NG, Jenkins NA, Nathans J (1996) Fibroblast growth factor (FGF) homologous factors: New members of the FGF family implicated in nervous system development. Proc Natl Acad Sci U S A 93:9850–9857

Sorokin A, Mohammadi M, Huang J, Schlessinger J (1994) Internalization of fibroblast growth factor receptor is inhibited by a point mutation at tyrosine 766. J Biol Chem 269:17056–17061

Spivak-Kroizman T, Lemmon MA, Dikic I, Ladbury JE, Pinchasi D, Huang J, Jaye M, Crumley G, Schlessinger J, Lax I (1994) Heparin-induced oligomerization of FGF molecules is responsible for FGF receptor dimerization, activation, and cell proliferation. Cell 79:1015–1024

Stachowiak MK, Moffett J, Joy A, Puchacz E, Florkiewicz R, Stachowiak EK (1994) Regulation of bFGF gene expression and subcellular distribution of bFGF protein in adrenal medullary cells. J Cell Biol 127:203–223

Stauber DJ, DiGabriele AD, Hendrickson WA (2000) Structural interactions of fibroblast growth factor receptor with its ligands. Proc Natl Acad Sci U S A 97:49–54

Steegmaier M, Levinovitz A, Isenmann S, Borges E, Lenter M, Kocher HP, Kleuser B, Vestweber D (1995) The E-selectin-ligand ESL-1 is a variant of a receptor for fibroblast growth factor. Nature 373:615–620

Szebenyi G Fallon JF (1999) Fibroblast growth factors as multifunctional signaling factors. Int Rev Cytol 185:45–106

Tanaka A, Miyamoto K, Minamino N, Takeda M, Sato B, Matsuo H, Matsumoto K (1992) Cloning and characterization of an androgen-induced growth factor essential for the androgen-dependent growth of mouse mammary carcinoma cells. Proc Natl Acad Sci U S A 89:8928–8932

Tarantini F, LaVallee T, Jackson A, Gamble S, Mouta CC, Garfinkel S, Burgess WH, Maciag T (1998) The extravesicular domain of synaptotagmin-1 is released with the latent fibroblast growth factor-1 homodimer in response to heat shock. J Biol Chem 273:22209–22216

Ueno H, Gunn M, Dell K, Tseng A, Jr., Williams L (1992) A truncated form of fibroblast growth factor receptor 1 inhibits signal transduction by multiple types of fibroblast growth factor receptor. J Biol Chem 267:1470–1476

Vagner S, Gensac MC, Maret A, Bayard F, Amalric F, Prats H, Prats AC (1995) Alternative translation of human fibroblast growth factor 2 mRNA occurs by internal entry of ribosomes. Mol Cell Biol 15:35–44

Vagner S, Touriol C, Galy B, Audigier S, Gensac MC, Amalric F, Bayard F, Prats H, Prats AC (1996) Translation of CUG- but not AUG-initiated forms of human fibroblast growth factor 2 is activated in transformed and stressed cells. J Cell Biol 135:1391–1402

Vainikka S, Joukov V, Klint P, Alitalo K (1996) Association of a 85-kDa serine kinase with activated fibroblast growth factor receptor-4. J Biol Chem 271:1270–1273

Van den BL, Laurell H, Huez I, Zanibellato C, Prats H, Bugler B (2000) FIF [fibroblast growth factor-2 (FGF-2)-interacting-factor], a nuclear putatively antiapoptotic factor, interacts specifically with FGF-2. Mol Endocrinol 14:1709–1724 van Deurs B, Petersen OW, Olsnes S, Sandvig K (1989) The ways of endocytosis. Int Rev Cytol 117:131–177

van Heumen WR, Claxton C, Pickles JO (1999) Fibroblast growth factor receptor-4 splice variants cause deletion of a critical tyrosine. IUBMB Life 48:73–78

Vasiliauskas D Stern CD (2001) Patterning the embryonic axis: FGF signaling and how vertebrate embryos measure time. Cell 106:133–136

Wang Q, McEwen DG, Ornitz DM (2000) Subcellular and developmental expression of alternatively spliced forms of fibroblast growth factor 14. Mech Dev 90:283–287

Welm BE, Freeman KW, Chen M, Contreras A, Spencer DM, Rosen JM (2002) Inducible dimerization of FGFR1: Development of a mouse model to analyze progressive transformation of the mammary gland. J Cell Biol 157:703–714

Werner S, Peters KG, Longaker MT, Fuller-Pace F, Banda MJ, Williams LT (1992) Large induction of keratinocyte growth factor expression in the dermis during wound healing. Proc Natl Acad Sci U S A 89:6896–6900

Wesche J, Wiedlocha A, Falnes PO, Choe S, Olsnes S (2000) Externally added aFGF mutants do not require extensive unfolding for transport to the cytosol and the nucleus in NIH/3T3 cells. Biochemistry 39:15091–15100

Wiedlocha A, Falnes PO, Madshus IH, Sandvig K, Olsnes S (1994) Dual mode of signal transduction by externally added acidic fibroblast growth factor. Cell 76:1039–1051

Wiedlocha A, Falnes PO, Rapak A, Klingenberg O, Munoz R, Olsnes S (1995) Translocation of cytosol of exogenous, CAAX-tagged acidic fibroblast growth factor. J Biol Chem 270:30680–30685

Wiedlocha A, Falnes PO, Rapak A, Munoz R, Klingenberg O, Olsnes S (1996) Stimulation of proliferation of a human osteosarcoma cell line by exogenous acidic fibroblast growth factor requires both activation of receptor tyrosine kinase and growth factor internalization. Mol Cell Biol 16:270–280

Wong A, Lamothe B, Lee A, Schlessinger J, Lax I, Li A (2002) FRS2 alpha attenuates FGF receptor signaling by Grb2-mediated recruitment of the ubiquitin ligase Cbl. Proc Natl Acad Sci U S A 99:6684–6689

Wright JA Huang A (1996) Growth factors in mechanisms of malignancy: roles for TGF-beta and FGF. Histol Histopathol 11:521–536

Wu ZL, Zhang L, Yabe T, Kuberan B, Beeler DL, Love A, Rosenberg RD (2003) The involvement of heparan sulfate (HS) in FGF1/HS/FGFR1 signaling complex. J Biol Chem 278:17121–17129

Yan G, McBride G, McKeehan WL (1993) Exon skipping causes alteration of the COOH-terminus and deletion of the phospholipase C gamma 1 interaction site in the FGF receptor 2 kinase in normal prostate epithelial cells. Biochem Biophys Res Commun 194:512–518

Yao H, York RD, Misra-Press A, Carr DW, Stork PJ (1998) The cyclic adenosine monophosphate-dependent protein kinase (PKA) is required for the sustained activation of mitogen-activated kinases and gene expression by nerve growth factor. J Biol Chem 273:8240–8247

Yayon A, Klagsbrun M, Esko JD, Leder P, Ornitz DM (1991) Cell surface, heparin-like molecules are required for binding of basic fibroblast growth factor to its high affinity receptor. Cell 64:841–848

Yayon A, Ma YS, Safran M, Klagsbrun M, Halaban R (1997) Suppression of autocrine cell proliferation and tumorigenesis of human melanoma cells and fibroblast growth factor transformed fibroblasts by a kinase-deficient FGF receptor 1: Evidence for the involvement of Src-family kinases. Oncogene 14:2999–3009

Yeh BK, Igarashi M, Eliseenkova AV, Plotnikov AN, Sher I, Ron D, Aaronson SA, Mohammadi M (2003) Structural basis by which alternative splicing confers specificity in fibroblast growth factor receptors. Proc Natl Acad Sci U S A 100:2266–2271

Yu K Ornitz DM (2001) Uncoupling fibroblast growth factor receptor 2 ligand binding specificity leads to Apert syndrome-like phenotypes. Proc Natl Acad Sci U S A 98:3641–3643

Zhan X, Hu X, Friesel R, Maciag T (1993) Long term growth factor exposure and differential tyrosine phosphorylation are required for DNA synthesis in BALB/c 3T3 cells. J Biol Chem 268:9611–9620

Zhan X, Plourde C, Hu X, Friesel R, Maciag T (1994) Association of fibroblast growth factor receptor-1 with c-Src correlates with association between c-Src and cortactin. J Biol Chem 269:20221–20224

Zhang JD, Cousens LS, Barr PJ, Sprang SR (1991) Three-dimensional structure of human basic fibroblast growth factor, a structural homolog of interleukin 1 beta. Proc Natl Acad Sci U S A 88:3446–3450

Zhou Z, Zuber ME, Burrus LW, Olwin BB (1997) Identification and characterization of a fibroblast growth factor (FGF) binding domain in the cysteine-rich FGF receptor. J Biol Chem 272:5167–5174

Zhu X, Komiya H, Chirino A, Faham S, Fox GM, Arakawa T, Hsu BT, Rees DC (1991) Three-dimensional structures of acidic and basic fibroblast growth factors. Science 251:90–93

Zuber ME, Zhou Z, Burrus LW, Olwin BB (1997) Cysteine-rich FGF receptor regulates intracellular FGF-1 and FGF-2 levels. J Cell Physiol 170:217–227

Zuniga Mejia BA, Meijers C, Zeller R (1993) Expression of alternatively spliced bFGF first coding exons and antisense mRNAs during chicken embryogenesis. Dev Biol 157:110–118

CTMI (2004) 286:81–118
© Springer-Verlag 2004

Ubiquitin System-Dependent Regulation of Growth Hormone Receptor Signal Transduction

G. J. Strous (✉) · C. Alves dos Santos · J. Gent · R. Govers · M. Sachse · J. Schantl · P. van Kerkhof

Department of Cell Biology, University Medical Center Utrecht
and Institute of Biomembranes, Heidelberglaan 100, AZU-G02.525,
3584 CX Utrecht, The Netherlands
strous@med.uu.nl

Abstract The growth hormone (GH) receptor is a key regulator of cellular metabolism. Unlike most growth factor receptors, its downregulation is not initiated by its ligand. Like many growth factor receptors, specific molecular mechanisms guarantee that a receptor can signal only once in its lifetime. Three features render the GH receptor unique: (a) an active ubiquitination system is required for both uptake (endocytosis) and degradation in the lysosomes; (b) uptake of the receptor is a continuous process, *independent* of both GH binding and Jak2 signal transduction; (c) only the cell surface expression of *dimerised* GH receptors is controlled by the ubiquitin system. This system enables two independent regulatory mechanisms for the endocrinology of the GH/GHR axis: the pulsatile secretion of GH by the pituitary and the GH sensitivity of individual cells of the body by the effects of the ubiquitin system on GH receptor availability.

Abbreviations

AP2   Heterotetrameric adaptor protein complex 2
CIS   Cytokine-inducible SH2 domain-containing protein
EGF   Epidermal growth factor
EpoR Erythropoietin receptor
ER   Endoplasmic reticulum
GH   Growth hormone
GHR   Growth hormone receptor
IGF   Insulin-like growth factor
IRS   Insulin receptor substrate
LDL   Low-density lipoprotein
LRP   LDL receptor-related protein
NGF   Nerve growth factor
PDGF Platelet-derived growth factor
RTK   Receptor tyrosine kinase
SE   Sorting endosome
SH2   Src homology 2
SOCS Suppressor of cytokine signalling
STAT Signal transducer and activator of transcription
TfR   Transferrin receptor
TMD   Transmembrane domain

1
Introduction

For a long time, the predominant view on the effectiveness of growth factor receptors was linear: Gene expression regulation determines the number of growth factor receptors at the cell surface, whereas their ligands, the growth factors, delimit timing and intensity of signal transduction. A regulatory potential of receptor control and involvement of intracellular compartments was hardly appreciated. Although gene expression levels (mRNA concentrations) are principally important, recent discoveries reveal signalling scenarios which implicate the full extent of the vacuolar system and the surprising picture emerges that, once translated, receptors are regulated individually. For some receptors protein folding, quality control, oligomerisation and protein complex formation in the endoplasmic reticulum (ER) determine their cell surface expression; for others, ligand-induced endocytosis is a major signal transduction regulator. Selective molecular mechanisms at endosomes appear to be another important determinant in signalling capacity: They can either send the receptors back to the cell surface for prolonged signalling or route them towards the lysosomes for destruction. In addition, specific locations can affect the signalling initiated at the cell surface, e.g. by attenuating, boosting or changing signalling pathways. Growth factor receptor signalling is not linear: Signals generated by one receptor can affect and activate other receptors both at the cell surface and in endosomes. In other scenarios proteolytic events convert portions of receptors into factors involved in DNA transcription. For the growth hormone receptor (GHR), cell surface expression and signalling modes are not less complex. The receptor has an extremely rapid turnover, dictated by the activity of the ubiquitin system, not by its ligand, the growth hormone (GH). All organelles of the vacuolar system are involved in its life and death, rendering it a textbook example.

This review discusses recent studies which have uncovered different determinants in the signalling of the GHR. The major focus is on the involvement of the ubiquitin conjugation system in the fate of the receptor. From various studies in yeast, consensus emerges that nutrient-regulated permeases depend on ubiquitination by the ubiquitin ligase Rsp5p for their degradation. In mammalian cells, several activated receptor tyrosine kinases (RTKs), such for epidermal growth factor (EGF), the hepatocyte growth factor, and platelet-derived growth factor (PDGF), depend on the ubiquitin ligase c-Cbl for their lysosomal degradation. In fact, the GHR is the only well-documented growth factor receptor whose removal from the cell surface depends on an active ubiquitination machinery. Unique in this event is that it is ligand independent. As for the RTKs, an equally important sorting step in controlling the signalling potential occurs at the level of the sorting endosomes (SEs). The GHR and its ligand GH are of basic importance for regulation of metabolism in humans, and therefore its cell biology must be carefully and precisely regulated.

2
GHR Traffic Control

2.1
The GHR

GH regulates postnatal growth as well as lipid and carbohydrate metabolism (Isaksson et al. 1985). Hyposecretion results in dwarfism, whereas hypersecretion leads to gigantism, a clinical condition known as acromegaly. The secretion of GH is regulated by a complex neuroendocrine system which involves both neural and feedback regulatory components. At least two hypothalamic hormones, a stimulatory GH-releasing hormone and an inhibitory hormone, somatostatin, generate a striking pulsatile pattern of GH release (Miller et al. 1982). Experimental animal studies have established that both growth and metabolic actions depend on the pattern of GH exposure, indicating that signalling is concentration- and time dependent (Jansson et al. 1982). Influences of gender, body composition and exercise play important roles in influencing circulating GH concentrations; secretion declines during normal aging, and many age-related changes, including osteoporosis and muscle atrophy, may be due, in part, to the decreased actions of GH and insulin-like growth factor 1 (IGF-1) (Casanueva 1992).

GH effects are mediated via the GHR, a member of the class I cytokine receptor superfamily which in addition includes the receptors for erythropoietin (Epo), prolactin, thrombopoietin, leptin, ciliary neurotropic factor, leukaemia inhibitory factor, granulocyte colony-stimulating factor and several of the interleukins. Although the overall homology between the members is low, some conserved motifs have been identified (reviewed in Bazan 1990). Their extracellular domain contains two or three pairs of disulfide-linked cysteine residues and a WSXWS (Trp, Ser, any amino acid, Trp, Ser) motif, which is indirectly involved in ligand binding (Carter-Su et al. 1996). The structure of the GHR is depicted in Fig. 1.

Strong proof for the functional significance of the GHR came from the demonstration of splice defects in the extracellular region of the GHR in patients with Laron syndrome (Godowski et al. 1989). This form of dwarfism, which is characterised by inherited GH insensitivity syndrome, was identified by Laron et al. and has a clinical phenotype of severe growth retardation with high circulating GH accompanied by low serum IGF-1 and IGF-binding protein-3, with no responsiveness to exogenous GH (Laron et al. 1966). In the inherited GH insensitivity syndrome, over 30 mutations in the GHR have been described, with the majority of the mutations in the exons which code for the extracellular domain of the receptor, interfering with GH binding (Rosenbloom 2000; Ross 1999). Recently, a heterozygous point mutation in the splice acceptor site, upstream of exon 9, was described. This mutation resulted in exon 9 being omitted from the GHR mRNA, creating a truncated receptor GHR(1–277) with only seven residues in the intracellular domain (Ayling et al. 1999; Iida et al. 1999). This receptor does bind GH but is unable to transmit the signal to the downstream signalling pathway. Al-

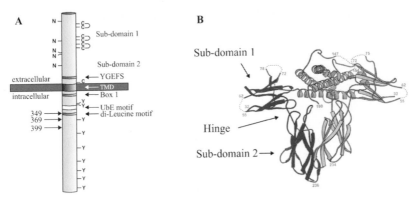

Fig. 1. A Schematic representation of the GHR. The GHR is a type I membrane protein (620 amino acid residues) and consists of an extracellular domain (246 aa), a single transmembrane domain (24 aa, *TMD*) and a cytoplasmic region (350 aa). The extracellular domain contains potential N-linked glycosylation sites (*N*), cysteine residues (*C*) and a WSxWS motif (in rabbit GHR: YGEFS) at the indicated positions. In the cytoplasmic domain, box 1, a proline-rich region required for signalling, and the ubiquitin-dependent endocytosis (*UbE*) and the di-leucine motifs are shown. Furthermore, rabbit GHR contains nine intracellular tyrosine residues, which are possibly involved in signalling. *Numbers to the left* indicate truncation mutants that are discussed in the text. **B** Structure of the GH-(GHR)2 complex. Ribbon rendering of the complex of one GH molecule and two GHR extracellular domains (shown in *dark and light grey*) (de Vos et al. 1992). The four α-helical bundle GH is seen at the *top* of the complex. The GHR extracellular domain is composed of two fibronectin type III domains (sub-domains 1 and 2), each consisting of seven β-strands. A four-amino acid hinge region separates the two sub-domains. (Adapted from de Vos et al. 1992)

ternative splices of the GHR, resulting in truncated isoforms, were identified in a permanent cell line of IM-9 cells and in a number of human tissues (Dastot et al. 1996, Ross et al. 1997). The alternative splices represented less than 10% of the total transcripts and are believed to act as dominant-negative inhibitors of GHR signalling by heterodimerisation with the full-length wild-type receptor [GHR(1–620)]. These findings suggest that differential expression of GHR isoforms could play a significant role in GHR signalling.

All cytokine receptors lack intrinsic kinase activity. Instead, they contain a cytosolic proline-rich domain, box 1, which functions as a binding site for members of the family of Jak2 tyrosine kinases. In the case of GHR, ligand binding leads to tyrosine phosphorylation of Jak2, the receptor and downstream signalling molecules (reviewed in Argetsinger et al. 1993).

2.2
GHR Dimerisation and Traffic Control in the ER

On the basis of crystallographic data, it was postulated that a single GH molecule dimerises two GHR molecules through interactions between the membrane proximal extracellular regions of adjacent GHR molecules, referred to as sub-domain 2 (de Vos et al. 1992) (Fig. 1B). Mutations of conserved amino acids in this domain disrupt ligand-induced signal transduction, presumably by conformational changes rather than by preventing receptor dimerisation (Gent et al. 2002, Chen et al. 1997). However, dimerisation itself is not sufficient for signal transduction because administration of monoclonal antibodies directed against the extracellular domain of the GHR resulted in dimerised GHRs but failed to induce signal transduction. The GHR extracellular domain contains two sub-domains, which are separated by a hinge region (Fig. 1B) (de Vos et al. 1992). Mellado et al. who developed a monoclonal antibody against the extracellular hinge region of the GHR (Mellado et al. 1997), showed that antibody binding to the cell surface receptor increased upon GH binding, but not when the GH antagonist GH (G120R), mutated in the second GHR binding domain, was used. This suggests that signal transduction requires a specific orientation of two GHR molecules. In recent years, evidence has accumulated that GHR already exists as a pre-formed dimer at the cell surface. Cross-linking studies with ^{125}I-GH or GH antagonist revealed complexes similar in size which correspond to a GH-(GHR)$_2$ complex (Harding et al. 1996, van Kerkhof et al. 2002). Conclusive evidence was provided by the finding that immunoprecipitation of a full-length GHR resulted in co-immunoprecipitation of a truncated receptor which was not recognised by the antibody used in the immunoprecipitation (Gent et al. 2002). This interaction most likely reflects dimerisation, as larger complexes, containing more than two GHR molecules, have not been observed. Strikingly, dimerisation was not only observed between mature, glycosylated forms of the receptor but also between precursor species, which reside in the ER. These findings indicate that receptor dimerisation already occurs in the ER and is independent of ligand binding. The molecular mechanism of GHR dimerisation in the ER is still unknown, but there are indications that neither the transmembrane domain (TMD) nor the cytosolic domain of the receptor is involved in dimerisation. Elimination of 97% of the cytoplasmic tail of the GHR does not effect the heterodimerisation of the truncated GHR with full-length GHR (Ross et al. 1997). Furthermore, mutating single and multiple amino acids of the TMD to alanine or replacement of the GHR TMD by a heterologous TMD does not disrupt GHR dimerisation (Gent and Strous, unpublished data), thereby rendering the extracellular domain an important player in receptor dimerisation. A role for the extracellular domain in the dimerisation process was suggested because replacement of the entire extracellular domain with part of the LDL receptor-related protein (LRP) results in monomeric chimers (Gent et al. 2003, Gent et al. 2002). On the other hand, the extracellular domain is not required to maintain the GHR in the dimerised state, because, once dimerised, protease digestion of the cell surface-localised GHRs does not disrupt dimerisation of the membrane-bound remnant protein. Therefore, the extracellular domain might be involved in the initial dimerisation process in the ER, whereas the TMD could be sufficient to maintain the GHR dimerised. A model of GHR dimerisation is shown in Fig. 2.

Although GH is not required for dimerisation , GH binding is essential for signal transduction. The activation of GHRs upon GH binding probably results in a conformational change of the receptor complex, leading to signal transduction events inside the cell. Mutations of amino acids of sub-domain 2 prevent the reorganisation induced by GH and result in signalling-deficient mutants without interfering with GHR

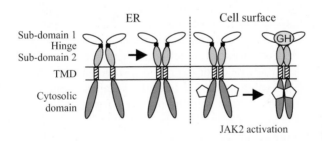

Fig. 2. GHR dimerisation in the ER and GH-induced activation at the cell surface. Dimerisation of GHRs occurs in the ER and is maintained during transport to the cell surface. The GHR extracellular domain is composed of an N-terminal GH binding sub-domain 1 and the membrane-proximal sub-domain 2, which can interact with sub-domain 2 of an adjacent GHR. ER chaperones facilitate this dimerisation. A hinge region separates the two domains. The TMDs of the dimerized GHRs are likely to be involved in stabilisation of the dimers. At the cell surface, GH binding induces a conformational change in the GHR-dimer, resulting in recruitment and cross-activation of two Jak2 tyrosine kinase molecules

dimerisation (Gent et al. 2003). These results link sub-domain 2 to signal transduction rather than dimerisation (Fig. 2). For various membrane proteins ligand-independent oligomerisation has also been reported. As has been demonstrated for the erythropoietin receptor (EpoR) (Constantinescu et al. 2001, Remy et al. 1999), EGF-R (Martin-Fernandez et al. 2002, Moriki et al. 2001) and melatonin receptor 1 and 2 (Ayoub et al. 2002), these preformed complexes are activated through a ligand-induced conformational change.

Once dimerised, it is likely that GHR receptors stay associated during transport to the cell surface. The presence of GHR dimers at the plasma membrane offers an advantage for rapid signalling. First, low ligand concentrations might still be able to initiate receptor signalling, which is especially advantageous in cells with low GHR levels; second, no time is lost in recruiting a second receptor to the GH-GHR complex (Cunningham et al. 1991).

Except for homo-dimerisation, the ER does not seem to play a role in GHR surface expression. Pulse-chase experiments showed that most, if not all, of the GHR initially synthesised in the ER matures into complex-glycosylated 130-kDa polypeptides. Use of proteasom inhibitors to prevent degradation of mal-folded intermediates did not change the amounts of precursor and mature GHRs, nor did they effect the maturation rate of the GHR (van Kerkhof et al. 2000a). Thus the ER does not seem to play a regulatory role in the expression of GHR at the cell surface. This is in distinct contrast to the situation for another important cytokine receptor, the EpoR. The N-terminal 32–58 residues of the JH7 domain of Jak2, not of Jak1, bind to the EpoR in the ER and promote its cell surface expression. A continuous stretch of amino acids in the EpoR cytosolic tail is required for functional, ligand-independent binding to Jak2 and cell surface receptor expression, whereas four specific residues are essential in switching on pre-bound Jak2 after ligand binding. Thus, in addition to its kinase activity required for cytokine receptor signalling, Jak2 is also an essential subunit required for surface expression of EpoR (Huang, et al. 2001). No role for Jak2 in ER to Golgi transport of the GHR was obvious from experiments with Jak2$^{-/-}$ mouse embryonic fibroblasts in which we expressed the GHR (Alves dos Santos and Strous, unpublished observation).

2.3
GHR Traffic Control at the Plasma Membrane

At the cell surface the expression of GHR is controlled by two major factors: (a) endocytosis and (b) proteolytic cleavage of the extracellular domain. In the first process the clathrin-mediated endocytosis of the GHR depends on the activity of the ubiquitin system, and the second factor is theactivity of tumour necrosis factor-α-converting enzyme (TACE), also referred to as Adam17. Together, they determine for more than 90% the residence time of the GHR at the cell surface. Inhibition of both activities prolongs the half-life of the GHR from less than 1 h to several hours. Thus inhibition of both GHR endocytosis and degradation at the cell surface renders the cells several-fold more sensitive for GH (van Kerkhof et al. 2003).

In a Chinese hamster cell line (ts20) with a temperature-sensitive mutation in the ubiquitin-activating enzyme E1, expressing the wild-type GHR, it was shown that endocytosis and degradation of the GHR are dependent on a functional ubiquitin conjugation system. Poly-ubiquitination of the GHR is enhanced upon binding of GH at the permissive temperature and completely inhibited at the non-permissive temperature (Strous et al. 1996). Examination of truncated receptors, the endocytosis-deficient receptor mutant F327A, and conditions under which clathrin-mediated endocytosis is inhibited shows that GHR ubiquitination and internalisation are coupled events (Govers et al. 1997). Surprisingly, the internalisation of a truncated receptor, GHR (1–399; K271–362R), which is not ubiquitinated because all cytoplasmic lysine residues (i.e. the acceptor sites for ubiquitin) are replaced with arginine residues, still depends on a functional ubiquitin conjugation system (Govers et al. 1999).

A specific domain in the GHR cytoplasmic tail regulates receptor endocytosis via the ubiquitin conjugation system. This domain, the ubiquitin-dependent endocytosis motif (UbE motif), consists of the amino acid sequence DSWVEFIELD (Govers et al. 1999). In addition to the UbE motif, the cytoplasmic tail of the GHR contains a di-leucine motif at position 347. Upon truncation of the receptor at amino acid residue 349, this di-leucine motif is exposed and mediates ubiquitin-system-*independent* internalisation of the GHR. Similar to wtGHR, di-leucine-mediated GHR internalisation requires functional clathrin-coated pits and results in GHR transport to the lysosome. However, the full-length GHR internalises independent of the di-leucine motif (Govers et al. 1998).

The ubiquitin-proteasome degradation pathway provides the major pathway for non-lysosomal degradation (reviewed in Hershko and Ciechanover 1998). It is involved in the degradation of cytoplasmic proteins and proteins, which do not pass the quality control of the ER, and plays a role in regulating a variety of cellular functions (Plemper and Wolf 1999). Degradation is initiated by the ubiquitin conjugation system, through which poly-ubiquitin moieties are attached to cytoplasmic proteins, after which the modified proteins are recognised and degraded by a multi-subunit protease, the 26S proteasome (Thrower et al. 2000). Recently, it became evident that for a restricted number of plasma membrane proteins, ubiquitination triggers internalisation and vacuolar/lysosomal rather than proteasomal degradation (reviewed in Strous and Govers 1999). This pathway is best understood in yeast, where a number of plasma membrane proteins is endocytosed in an ubiquitin-dependent manner (Galan et al. 1996; Hicke 2001; Kölling and Hollenberg 1994; Terrell et al. 1998).

Endocytosis of the GHR occurs via the clathrin-mediated pathway but is regulated via the ubiquitin-proteasome system (Strous and van Kerkhof 2002) and requires an intact UbE motif (Govers et al. 1999). The formation of clathrin-coated pits at the plasma membrane and the recruitment of cargo proteins involve a network of proteins called adaptors, which mediate binding between cargo proteins and clathrin. Adaptors in clathrin-coated pit formation at the plasma membrane are (a) monomeric arrestins and (b) the heterotetrameric adaptor complex 2 (AP2). Non-visual arrestins are involved in the internalisation of a number of G protein-coupled receptors. For example, after ligand stimulation, the activated β2-adrenergic receptor is recruited by β-arrestin into clathrin-coated pits (Goodman et al. 1996, Santini et al. 2002). β-Arrestin can bind with its C-terminus to clathrin as well as to AP2 (Krupnick et al. 1997, Laporte et al. 1999). It was therefore suggested that the interaction with AP2 is required to cluster the β2-adrenergic receptor in clathrin-coated pits (Laporte et al. 2000).

The heterotetrameric adaptor complex AP2 belongs to a family of adaptor complexes consisting of AP1, AP2, AP3 and AP4 (for review see Kirchhausen 1999). All these complexes consist of two large subunits of about 100–130 kDa (α and β2 in AP2), a central subunit of 50 kDa (μ2 in AP2) and a small subunit around 20 kDa (σ2 in AP2). At the plasma membrane AP2 can function as a bridge between cargo membrane proteins and the clathrin coat. The interaction with clathrin is mediated by its β2 subunit and was narrowed down to a so-called "clathrin box", which is conserved amongst a number of clathrin-interacting proteins

(Gallusser and Kirchhausen 1993, Terhaar et al. 2000). Correct trafficking of membrane proteins depends on signal sequences or sorting signals. Interaction of cargo with AP2 generally depends on the presence of short peptide motifs of four to six amino acid residues present in the cytoplasmic tail (reviewed in Bonifacino and Traub, 2003).

The first sorting signal required for endocytosis was identified in the LDL receptor and consists of a peptide NPXY (X representing any amino acid). This motif is necessary and sufficient to mediate endocytosis (Chen et al. 1990) and interacts with the µ2 subunit of AP2 (Boll et al. 2002). More widely used is the YXXØ motif (Ø stands for a bulky hydrophobic side chain), which was first identified in the transferrin receptor (TfR) (Collawn et al. 1990). Support for the idea that YXXØ motifs interact with AP2 came from studies in which ligand-stimulated EGF-R coimmunoprecipitated AP2; this interaction depended on the presence of the YXXØ motif (Sorkin and Carpenter 1993; Sorkin et al. 1996). In yeast-two hybrid screens, it was shown that YXXØ motifs interact with the µ2 subunit of AP2 (Ohno et al. 1995). For the interaction of the µ2 subunit with EGF-R, the amino acid residues D176 and W421 of µ2 are crucial. Also, for TfR internalisation interaction with AP2 via the µ2 subunit is a pre-requisite. For the chicken GHR an interaction between α-adaptin and the GHR has been shown upon hormone stimulation (Vleurick et al. 1999). Considering that GH triggers neither mouse nor rabbit GHR endocytosis, this observation is in line with our observations that GHR endocytosis is K^+ dependent and that only endocytosis-competent GHR is present in clathrin-coated pits by immunogold electron microscopy (Govers et al. 1997, Sachse et al. 2001). However, attempts to find an association between AP2 and GHR failed, probably because of competition between factors of the ubiquitin system and AP2 (Schantl and Strous, unpublished data). In other membrane cargo proteins, for example, the CI-MPR and CD4, acidic di-leucine motifs mediate endocytosis (Glickman et al. 1989, Shin et al. 1991). This motif binds to the β2 subunit of AP2 (Rapoport et al. 1998). Proteins containing this motif do not compete in vivo for endocytic uptake with those containing a YXXØ motif, suggesting that they use distinct pathways, both depending on AP2 (Marks et al. 1997).

In the past few years, it has been demonstrated for an increasing number of yeast plasma membrane proteins that ubiquitination is required for their internalisation. Several studies showed that mono-ubiquitination of proteins is sufficient to stimulate their endocytosis (Galan and Haguenauer-Tsapis 1997; Roth and Davis 2000; Terrell et al. 1998). In mammalian cells, the GHR, the β-adrenergic receptor and the epithelial sodium channel, ENaC, are the only cell surface proteins known which endocytose ubiquitin system-dependently (Shenoy et al. 2001; Staub et al. 1997; Strous and Gent 2002). Ubiquitin itself contains none of the above-mentioned sorting signals. Moreover, no ubiquitin moiety needs to be attached to the GHR at the time of endocytosis (Govers et al. 1999), whereas GHR endocytosis is completely blocked if the ubiquitin-activating enzyme E1 is inactivated (Strous et al. 1996). In yeast, endocytosis can occur independent of the AP2 orthologue (Huang et al. 1999). Therefore, it was suggested that two surface patches on the folded ubiquitin contain the information for internalisation of the ubiquitinated protein and may mediate the binding to the adaptor protein Epsin to initiate endocytosis (Shih et al. 2002; Shih et al. 2000). In mammalian cells, ubiquitination of β-arrestin by the E3 Mdm2 is required for endocytosis of the β2-adrenergic receptor, suggesting that the ubiquitination of an adaptor protein triggers endocytosis (Shenoy et al. 2001). Recently, accessory proteins involved in the primary steps of endocytosis, Eps15, Eps15R and Epsin, all three of which can bind clathrin as well as AP2, were shown to be mono-ubiquitinated (Klapisz et al. 2002; Polo et al. 2002; van Delft et al. 1997). The ubiquitination of these proteins suggests a regulatory function of ubiquitin in the endocytic machinery. Recently, the small glutamine-rich tetratricopeptide repeat-containing protein (SGT) was identified as a possible co-factor in GHR trafficking (Schantl et al. 2003). In Fig. 3 an overview of membrane protein cargo trafficking is depicted.

Taken together, four features render the GHR unique compared with other receptors that signal from the cell surface:

1. *Recruitment of the GHR into the coated pits depends on an active ubiquitin system.* This feature determines the average residence time at the cell surface. There is ample evidence from many clinical studies that in stress conditions the number of GHRs is decreased, because of rapid endocytosis (Frank 2001). A key role for the ubiquitin system in GHR internalisation emerges from both genetic and molecular experiments showing that GHR molecules accumulate at the plasma membrane if the ubiquitin system is inhibited (Strous and Govers 1999). Moreover, GHR ubiquitination coincides with its recruitment into clathrin-coated pits (van Kerkhof et al. 2000b). Strikingly, ubiquitination of the GHR itself is not required because replacement of all lysine residues by arginines in the GHR cytosolic tail does not inhibit internalisation (Govers et al. 1999). We have identified the target of the ubiquitin system in the GHR cytosolic tail as a 10-amino acid-long sequence, DSWVEFIELD,

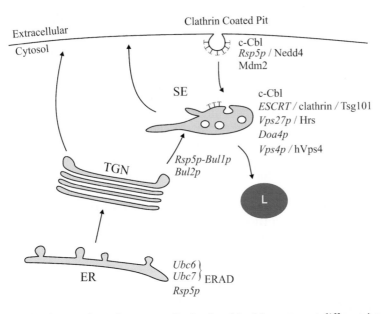

Fig. 3. Modulation of membrane proteins by the ubiquitin system at different intracellular locations. In the process of ER associated degradation (*ERAD*), malfolded proteins are recognized in the ER, translocated back into the cytosol, ubiquitinated (involving the E2 enzymes Ubc6 and Ubc7) and degraded by the 26S proteasome. At the *trans*-Golgi network the yeast HECT E3 Rsp5p acts together with Bul1p and Bul2p to direct the general amino acid permease (Gap1p) to a prevacuolar compartment [the yeast equivalent of the sorting endosome (*SE*)] instead of the plasma membrane (Soetens et al. 2001; Helliwell et al. 2001). Membrane proteins at the cell surface are often modified by covalent ubiquitin attachment. E3s involved in this process are indicated. Upon arrival in the SE, membrane proteins that have to be degraded in the vacuole/lysosome (*L*) are sorted away from proteins that recycle back to the plasma membrane. Sorting of cargo membrane proteins into the internal vesicles of the SE is mediated via the ubiquitin system and depends on the recognition of ubiquitinated proteins by proteins like Hrs, Tsg101 or the yeast ESCRT complex. Before inward budding is completed, ubiquitin moieties are removed from the ubiquitinated proteins by deubiquitinating enzymes such as yeast Doa4p, and the coat is disassembled by the AAA-ATPase Vps4p (Sachse et al. 2003). Finally, the membrane proteins are degraded by vacuolar or lysosomal protease. Yeast proteins are in *italics*

designated as the UbE motif for ubiquitin-dependent endocytosis (Govers et al. 1999). Besides the ubiquitin conjugating system, the 26S proteasome is also involved in GHR downregulation. Proteasome inhibitors prevent both internalisation of the GHR and endosome-to-lysosome transport (van Kerkhof et al. 2001; van Kerkhof et al. 2000a). The inhibitory effect is lost when the GHR is truncated beyond amino acid 369, suggesting that an associated protein must be degraded by the proteasome before internalisation can occur (Sachse et al. 2002; van Kerkhof et al. 2000b).

2. *Endocytosis of the GHR is constitutive and ligand independent.* Thus cell surface expression of the GHR is not regulated by its ligand; upon arrival at the cell surface from the ER/Golgi complex, the GHR is recruited into coated vesicles (like cargo receptors such as the LDL receptor) and transported to lysosomes for degradation (unlike cargo receptors, which release their cargo in endosomes and immediately return to the plasma membrane for the next round of endocytosis) (van Kerkhof et al. 2002). One exception to this rule constitutes the GHR in the human B-lymphoblast cell line IM-9. These cells show a GH accelerated receptor downregulation (Ilondo et al. 1986; Saito et al. 1994). Whether this is a feature induced by Epstein-Barr virus transformation, or by a mutation in the GHR gene, is unknown.

3. *Only dimerised GHR is recruited into the coated pits by the ubiquitin system.* Curiously, the UbE motif is only an effective ubiquitin system target if the GHR is in a dimeric state: Replacement of the GHR extracellular domain by a part of the extracellular domain of LRP prevents GHR dimerisation and disqualifies the ubiquitin system as a regulator of GHR endocytosis (Gent et al. 2002).

4. *The ubiquitin system regulates GH sensitivity of cells.* Until now only the interaction between the tumour suppressor p53 and the E3 Mdm2 seems to be a direct protein-protein interaction independent of phosphorylation, implying that the concentration of these proteins in cytosol and/or nucleus is a major factor in controlling cellular life and death. Whether availability of GHRs at the cell surface is subjected to the same kind of mechanism remains to be elucidated. There is a remarkable difference between the involvement of the ubiquitin system in GHR trafficking and in other membrane proteins: In most, if not all, systems reported, the activity of the ubiquitin system is preceded by protein phosphorylation. In yeast, uptake of Ste2p and most permeases requires phosphorylation of serine or threonine before action of Rsp5p initiates uptake (De Craene et al. 2001; Hicke et al. 1998). In mammalian cells, uptake of ENaC requires serine phosphorylation before the HECT domain of Nedd4 can bind to the tetrameric sodium channel. Degradation via the RING motif E3 βTrCP requires previous phosphorylation as documented for NFκB, β-catenin, HIV-1 protein vpu, cyclins and myo-D, whereas c-Cbl stimulates degradation of RTKs only if their kinase domain is active. As the signal transduction pathway of the GHR via Jak2 is not involved in ubiquitin system-dependent endocytosis

(Alves dos Santos et al. 2001), and no other phosphorylation event has ever been observed, it may be that GHR internalisation relies on the ubiquitination of a GHR-associated protein which either is constitutively phosphorylated or directs the GHR into the endocytic pathway in a phosphorylation-independent way.

2.4
GHR Traffic Control in Endosomes

Once recruited into a coated pit via factors of the ubiquitin system and endocytic machinery (e.g. AP2, Eps15, Epsin, clathrin, dynamin) the GHR becomes a cargo molecule in the early endosome (Fig. 3). At this point the system has two major options for cargo membrane proteins: (a) the default recycling route back to the cell surface and (b) a second sorting step for degradation in the lysosomes. The recycling pathway is common for receptors involved in uptake and scavenging of proteins from the circulation like LDL, asialoglycoproteins, α-macroglobulin and apo-E. These receptors (such as LDL receptor, asialoglycoprotein receptor, LRP) release their soluble cargo molecules in the acidic environment of the endosome (Yamashiro et al. 1984). The low pH is generated by the vacuolar ATPase and is crucial for sorting of ligands that show a pH-dependent affinity towards their receptors (Johnson et al. 1993, Schmid et al. 1989). The receptors return to the cell surface, while their cargo (ligands) remains in the lumen of the vacuole and is transported to lysosomes for degradation (Geuze et al. 1983). In the case of the TfR, the acidic pH causes iron to dissociate from the receptor ligand transferrin, after which the apoTf-TfR complex recycles to the plasma membrane (Dautry-Varsat et al. 1983; Klausner et al. 1983). For lysosomal degradation (option b) membrane proteins must be identified by the ESCRT system which is located in specialised coated membrane domains of the sorting endosomes (SEs) (Sachse et al. 2002). Among these cargo membrane proteins are many growth factor receptors whose ligand binding is stable at the lower pH values of the SE. A common localisation throughout the endocytic pathway was shown for EGF and EGF-R and, similarly, a pool of intact PDGF-PDGF-R and NGF-TrkA (nerve growth factor) receptor complexes could be detected in endosomes (Sorkin and Waters 1993). As sorting into the internal vesicles of SEs depends on several actors of the ubiquitin/proteasome system (discussed below), this step is easily inhibited by proteosome inhibitors. We have shown that the degradation of NGF, internalised via its receptor TrkA, is inhibited in the presence of proteasome inhibitors. Proteasome inhibitors were also shown to inhibit the degradation of the PDGF-R (Mori et al. 1995), the EGF-R (Levkowitz et al. 1998) and the Met tyrosine kinase receptor (Jeffers et al. 1997). RTKs are probably all sorted into the SE vesicles invaginating from the limiting membrane together with their ligands (Sachse et al. 2002). Also, for cytokine receptors it was indicated that proteasome inhibitors inhibit the downregulation at the SE (Martinez-Moczygemba and Huston 2001, Rocca et al. 2001; Verdier et al. 2000; Yen et al. 2000; Yu and Malek 2001). Notably, whereas membrane cargo proteins depend on ESCRT and the ubiquitin-proteasome system, soluble proteineous cargo and solutes travel via the same route by default (van Kerkhof et al. 2001).

Depending on the cell type, the vacuolar part of SEs is reached by endocytic tracers within 1–5 min (Kleijmeer et al. 1997; Schmid et al. 1988). By electron microscopy the irregularly shaped vacuole (250–500 nm) is electron-lucent with only a few internal vesicles. Internal endosomal vesicles are formed by inward budding of the limiting membrane, a process called micro-autophagy (Geuze 1998; Hopkins et al. 1990) (Fig. 3). In addition, SEs can bear a prominent clathrin coat (Holtzman and Dominitz 1968; Raposo et al. 2001; Sachse et al. 2002). Besides clathrin, coatomer complex I coats have been found on SEs, with a possible role in sorting of proteins towards lysosomal degradation (Gu et al. 1997; Piguet et al. 1999; Whitney et al. 1995).

The molecular mechanism for sorting the GHR into the SE internal vesicles remains largely unsolved. Unlike the RTKs, tyrosine kinase activity of recruited Jak2 is not required (Alves dos Santos et al. 2001). In RTKs both the ubiquitin ligase c-Cbl and the hepatocyte growth factor-regulated tyrosine kinase substrate Hrs act as intermediates in cargo selection by the ESCRT complex. For these events, the RTKs must be activated and the cytosolic tails must bear both phosphate residues and (mono)ubiquitin to accommodate the two factors. Hrs contains a clathrin-binding domain, localises to the flat clathrin lattices of SEs and binds directly to ubiquitin via its ubiquitin-interacting (UIM) motif (Raiborg et al. 2002; Sachse et al. 2002; Urbé et al. 2000; Urbé et al. 2003). GHR selection into the SE internal vesicles does not involve c-Cbl; it requires the general co-factors of ESCRT, Hrs and the AAA-type ATPase hVPS4 but does not require ubiquitination of the receptor (Govers et al. 1999; Sachse et al. 2003; van Kerkhof et al. 2001; van Kerkhof et al. 2000b).

The question then is, what is required for the GHR to pass the sorting step in the SE? As GHR endocytosis depends on a functional ubiquitin conjugation system, an intact UbE motif and active proteasomes, the answer is not easily obtained. Most of the experimental approaches use one of the three variables, conditions that inhibit GHR entry into the cells. To address this question, a GHR was truncated at position 349 of the cytosolic tail. In this truncated GHR a di-leucine motif is activated that mediates internalisation in an ubiquitin system- and proteasome-*independent* fashion (Govers et al. 1998). Mutation of phenylalanine residue 327 to alanine in the UbE motif abolished ubiquitination of both full length- and truncated GHR (Govers et al. 1999) but did not influence the internalisation of the truncated GHR(1–349). Both pulse chase and ^{125}I-GH uptake experiments showed that an intact UbE in the truncated GHR(1–349) is required for efficient degradation of both ligand and receptor (van Kerkhof et al. 2001). As the degradation of the ligand occurs in lysosomes (Murphy and Lazarus 1984; Yamada et al. 1987), the conclusion is that the UbE motif is required for endosome to lysosome sorting of both receptor and ligand and that the C-terminal di-leucine motif intermediary in endocytosis is not recognised by the cargo selectors at the SE. Thus the UbE motif is required both at the cell surface and at the SE for correct sorting and presumably the same factors of the ubiquitin conjugation system are involved. Analogous to the situation for EGF, PDGF and CSF-1 receptors, in which c-Cbl seems to initiate cargo selection at the SE by adding ubiquitin to the (phosphorylated) receptors (Joazeiro et al. 1999; Lee et al. 1999; Levkowitz et al. 1999; Miyake et al. 1998), all indications point to a ubiquitin ligase-specific for *dimerised* GHRs as initiator for cargo selection. The E3 for GHR sorting is unknown yet, but it is probably not c-Cbl as the GHR does not require GH-activation and Jak2 activity for this step. Very likely it will be the same E3 as required for GHR endocytosis. The E3-GHR complex might then be recognised by Hrs and incorporated into the ESCRT system. Whether ancillary factors are involved or other modifications are needed remains to be investigated. An interesting observation in this respect is that truncation of the cytosolic tail precedes degradation of the luminal domain (van Kerkhof and Strous 2001).

The idea that the same ubiquitination factors are involved at the cell surface and at the SE is strengthened by the observation that at both sites ubiquitination of the GHR per se is not needed, only competent cellular ubiquitination machinery and the UbE motif within the GHR cytosolic domain (Govers et al. 1999; van Kerkhof et al. 2001). This suggests that, in this system, ubiquitination of another component serves as cargo selection signal for the receptor, that ubiquitination and subsequent degradation of an inhibitory molecule promote exposure of a ubiquitin-independent sorting signal or that the docked ubiquitination machinery itself targets the complex for uptake. An example of the last possibility is the recent discovery that CIN85 bridges a receptor-bound E3 ligase and endophilin, a known endocytic protein, to promote internalisation (Petrelli et al. 2002; Soubeyran et al. 2002).

The involvement of proteasomes in the molecular mechanism of cargo packaging either at the cell surface or at the level of SEs is presently unclear. The half-life of many membrane proteins and growth factor receptors is increased twofold or more in the presence of proteasome inhibitors. We investigated the role of the ubiquitin-proteasome pathway in the degradation of GH and GHR(1–349) by using the peptide aldehyde MG-132 as well as the highly specific clasto-lactacystin β-lactone (Craiu et al. 1997). Under these conditions, GHR(1–349) can enter the cells freely via the di-leucine motif. Degradation of both the GH and the GHR(1–349) was almost completely inhibited, indicating that proteasome activity is required for sorting from the SE to the lysosome (van Kerkhof et al. 2001). Also, lysosomal sorting of NGF endocytosed via TrkA was completely inhibited by proteasome inhibitors, whereas endocytosis of TrkA does not depend on the ubiquitin-proteasome system. Again, this indicates that SE-to-lysosome transport requires the activity of the ubiquitin conjugation system, and perhaps also of the proteasome. It is possible that there is no direct role for the proteasome, because use of proteasome inhibitors might exhaust the cells of free ubiquitin which might lead to reduced ubiquitination of the target protein and reduced endosomal sorting (Swaminathan et al. 1999; van Kerkhof et al. 2001).

The question remains: What is the target for the proteasome? It is clear that shortly after endocytosis the degradation of the GHR starts at the cytosolic tail before it reaches the lysosomes (van Kerkhof and Strous 2001b). Whether this cytosolic degradation is due to proteasome activity remains unclear. A crucial question is whether cytosolic degradation is a requisite for cargo selection by the ubiquitin and the ESCRT system. The di-leucine motif probably does not play a role in this sorting event because its mutation does not affect the effective transport to lysosomes and degradation of GH (Govers et al. 1998). The conserved DSGRTS sequence between amino acid residues 365 and 370 is interesting, as similar sequences (consensus DSGxxS) in β-catenin and IκBα are targeted by specific kinases, after which the E3 βTrCP poly-ubiquitinates the two proteins (Aberle et al. 1997; Chen et al. 1995). Whether partial degradation of GHR plays a role in endosome to lysosome sorting via the DSGxxS motif remains to be investigated. A complicating factor is the observation that ubiquitination of the GHR is not required for proper sorting.

In conclusion, the data point to a specific role of the ubiquitin-proteasome pathway in the regulated sorting of specific sets of membrane proteins. On the basis of our observation that ubiquitination of the GHR itself is not required for this sorting, we speculate that a specific membrane protein recruits an ubiquitin ligase which then, directly or via ubiquitination of target proteins, recruits the sorting machinery to accomplish its subsequent degradation.

3
GHR Signalling Control

3.1
GH Binding to GHR

GH binding to the GHR is the first step in the signalling cascade. With crystallography and gel filtration, a single GH molecule was shown to form a ternary complex with two GHR extracellular domains (Cunningham et al. 1991; de Vos et al. 1992). Two distinct binding sites were found in GH: a high-affinity site 1 covering a surface area of about 1,230 $Å^2$ and a slightly lower-affinity site 2 of about 900 $Å^2$. Because of the different affinities, complex formation has been proposed to occur sequentially (Cunningham et al. 1991). Strikingly, the two distinct binding sites of GH interact with the same amino acids located in the N-terminal fibronectin type III domain (sub-domain 1) of the GHR molecules, suggesting that no more than one GH molecule can bind to a single GHR. Recruitment of the second GHR to the complex is a prerequisite for signal transduction as was demonstrated with a GH site 2 mutant. Mutation of the glycine at position 120 of human GH to arginine (G120R) or lysine (G120K) disrupts the binding via site 2 (Fuh et al. 1992). Because binding site 1 is unaffected, competition with endogenous GH for GHR molecules occurs, hence explaining the dwarf phenotype of transgenic mice overexpressing this GH site 2 mutant (Chen et al. 1990). In cell systems, the GH site 2 mutant antagonises the effects of GH when applied in a three to fivefold excess (Zhang et al. 1999). Combination of the G120K mutation with mutations which enhance the affinity of site 1 resulted in the potent GH antagonist B2036 (Maamra et al. 1999). When conjugated to polyethylene glycol to decrease glomerular

filtration in the kidney, this antagonist is effective in treatment of acro-
megalic patients (Trainer et al. 2000).

3.2
Signalling Events at the Cell Surface

GH binding to GHR induces the transcription of genes encoding for a
variety of proteins including GHR, IGF-1, insulin, LDL receptor, serine
protease inhibitor (spi) 2.1, cytochrome *P*450 and the transcription factors c-Fos, c-Jun and c-Myc (Carter-Su et al. 1996). The four known signalling pathways initiated by the GHR are depicted in Fig. 4. To initiate
signalling, GHR recruits and transiently activates the cytosolic tyrosine
kinase Jak2 (Argetsinger et al. 1993). This event takes place at the cell

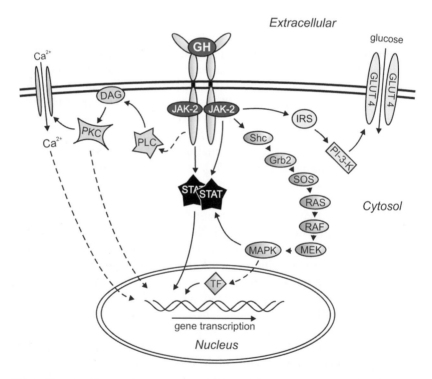

Fig. 4. The signalling pathways activated by GH. GH binding to GHR results in activation of the STAT, MAPK, IRS and/or PKC pathways which ultimately results in activation of gene transcription. See text for details. (Modified from Argetsinger and
Carter Su 1996)

surface because Jak2 is also activated by GH under conditions that impair GHR internalisation (potassium depletion) (Govers et al. 1997; Alves dos Santos et al. 2001). Mutation or deletion of the proline-rich box 1 region impairs Jak2 binding (Sotiropoulos et al. 1994; VanderKuur et al. 1994). However, for maximal Jak2 activation the membrane-proximal one-third of the GHR cytoplasmic domain is required. According to the current model, GH induces a conformational change in the dimerised GHR that brings two Jak2 molecules in close proximity, thereby facilitating trans-phosphorylation of tyrosine residues in the kinase domain of the paired Jak2 (Gent et al. 2002). Subsequently, these activated Jak2 molecules phosphorylate tyrosine residues of the GHR (Wang et al. 1996) and signalling molecules (Carter-Su et al. 1996). In general, phosphorylated tyrosine residues serve as docking sites for proteins with Src homology 2 (SH2) or phosphotyrosine binding domains.

A direct pathway from activated GHR to gene transcription involves members of the signal transducers and activators of transcription (STATs) family, the *STAT pathway* (Darnell 1997). STAT proteins are recruited via their SH2 domain to the phosphorylated GHR (e.g. STAT5A and -5B) or to Jak2 (e.g. STAT1 and -3), are then phosphorylated on a conserved C-terminal tyrosine residue, homo- or heterodimerise with other STAT molecules, translocate to the nucleus, bind to specific DNA promoter sequences and activate transcription of several target genes. For example, STAT1 and -3 bind to sis-inducible elements (SIE) in the c-Fos promoter (Campbell et al. 1995), whereas STAT5 binds the interferon-γ-activated sequence (GAS)-like response element (GLE) in the spi2.1 gene (Wood et al. 1997). Recently, the mitogen-activated protein (MAP) kinases ERK1 and ERK2 have been implicated in the serine phosphorylation of STAT proteins (Pircher et al. 1999). Both kinases are also activated in response to GH via a complex cascade known as the *RAS-MAP kinase pathway*. MAP kinases are serine/threonine kinases, which are activated by dual phosphorylation on tyrosine and threonine residues and are important regulators of cellular growth and differentiation (Cobb and Goldsmith 1995). The signalling pathway starts with the binding of the Src homology-containing (Shc) protein to activated Jak2, followed by Shc phosphorylation (VanderKuur et al. 1995). The cascade continues via growth factor receptor-bound 2 (Grb2), son of sevenless (SOS), RAS, RAF and mitogen-activated/extracellular signal-regulated kinase (MEK) and ultimately results in the activation of MAP kinases ERK1 and ERK2 (VanderKuur et al. 1997). In addition to the STAT pathway, MAP kinases activate a variety of proteins including phospholipase A2, the ribosomal S6 kinase p90RSK, cytoskeletal proteins and transcription factors like c-Jun, c-Myc and the ternary complex factor p62[TCF]/ELK1 (Davis 1993).

GH binding also results in the tyrosine phosphorylation of insulin receptor substrate (IRS)-1, IRS-2 and IRS-3 (Argetsinger et al. 1995; Souza et al. 1994). These molecules were identified as signalling molecules for insulin and the closely related IGFs and are therefore proposed to mediate the insulin-like effects (e.g. glucose uptake and lipogenesis) of GH. Phosphorylated IRS proteins associate with the 85-kDa regulatory subunit of phosphatidylinositol (PI)-3-kinase (Ridderstrale and Tornqvist 1994). PI-3-kinase activation leads to translocation of the insulin-dependent glucose transporter GLUT-4 to the plasma membrane, thereby stimulating the uptake of glucose (Cheatham et al. 1994). Consistently, inhibition of PI-3-kinase by wortmannin blocks the insulin-like effects of GH in rat adipocytes (Ridderstrale and Tornqvist 1994).

A fourth signalling pathway which is activated upon GH stimulation involves the activation of protein kinase C (PKC) through phospholipase C (PLC) (Moutoussamy et al. 1998). Although the exact mechanism of PLC activation is unknown, the involvement of a G protein has been suggested. Upon activation PLC hydrolyses inositol phospholipids to generate inositol phosphates and 1,2-diacylglycerol (DAG), which acts as a potent activator of PKC. The IRS/PI-3-kinase pathway has also been implicated in PKC activation, but this may be GH independent and restricted to certain PKC isoforms (Argetsinger and Carter Su 1996). Activated PKC stimulates lipogenesis and c-Fos expression and increases intracellular Ca^{2+} levels by activating L-type calcium channels (Gaur et al. 1996a, Gaur et al. 1996b). Intracellular calcium is essential for GH-induced transcription of the spi2.1 gene (Billestrup et al. 1995). Currently, regulation of Ca^{2+} influx via L-type calcium channels is the only event known which is Jak2 independent.

3.3
Modulation of Signal Transduction

In addition to the molecules initiating gene transcription, several factors have been proposed to modulate the GHR signalling activity. Phosphorylated Jak2 recruits the cytosolic SH2 domain-containing protein SH2-B, which stimulates the kinase activity of Jak2 and enhances signal transduction (Rui and Carter-Su 1999). Tyrosine phosphatases have been implicated in downregulation of GHR-mediated signalling. In response to GH, the SH2-domain containing tyrosine phosphatase SHP-1 binds and dephosphorylates Jak2 (Gebert et al. 1999; Hackett et al. 1997). Also

SHP-2, an ubiquitously expressed tyrosine phosphatase homologous to SHP-1, has been demonstrated to bind directly to a phosphorylated tyrosine residue in the C-terminal region of the GHR (Stofega et al. 2000). Mutation of this tyrosine residue or deletion of the C-terminal region results in the prolonged activation of the GHR, Jak2 and STAT5 (Alves dos Santos et al. 2001; Stofega et al. 2000). SHP-2 can also act via an ancillary protein: GH stimulation induces tyrosyl phosphorylation of the transmembrane glycoprotein signal-regulatory protein SIRPα1, which then recruits one or more SHP-2 molecules (Stofega et al. 1998). Interaction between SIRPα1 and SHP-2 enhances the phosphatase activity of SHP-2 and results in the dephosphorylation of SIRPα1, Jak2 and possibly the GHR (Stofega et al. 2000).

Recently, a new family of suppressor of cytokine signalling (SOCS) proteins has been implicated in a negative-feedback mechanism on cytokine signalling (Starr et al. 1997). In addition to a 40-amino acid C-terminal region called SOCS-box, all SOCS proteins contain a central SH2 domain (Krebs and Hilton 2000). Of the eight known members, GH induces rapid expression of SOCS-1, -2 and -3 and cytokine-inducible SH2-domain containing protein (CIS) to different extents (Adams et al. 1998; Tollet-Egnell et al. 1999), probably mediated via STAT proteins (Matsumoto et al. 1997). The importance of regulating signal transduction via SOCS proteins is demonstrated by the giant phenotype of mice lacking SOCS-2 (Metcalf et al. 2000) and the dwarf size when CIS is overexpressed (Matsumoto et al. 1999). The SOCS proteins use variable mechanisms to inhibit signalling. SOCS-1 inhibits Jak2 kinase activity by directly binding to the kinase activating domain (Yasukawa et al. 1999). SOCS-3 binds to tyrosine residues in close proximity to box 1 and might therefore prevent Jak2 association with the GHR (Ram and Waxman 1999). CIS and SOCS-2 bind to phosphotyrosine residues in the C-terminal region of GHR and compete with STATs and/or other signalling molecules (Ram and Waxman 1999). Recently, an alternative model has been proposed, based on the observation that the conserved SOCS-box binds to the elongin B/C complex (Zhang et al. 1999). These elongins also interact with cullin-2, a putative ubiquitin-ligase, and thereby mediate the ubiquitination and subsequent degradation of the SOCS protein and its interacting molecules like Jak2 (Ungureanu et al. 2002). Consistent with this model, proteasome inhibitors prolong phosphorylation of Jak2 and the GHR (Alves dos Santos et al. 2001).

3.4
Jak2 Activity and GHR Trafficking Are Independent

The role of Jak2-mediated signal transduction in GHR membrane trafficking seems to be minor. For the EpoR, another cytokine receptor, the regulation of cell surface expression depends on Jak2. Jak2, not Jak1, binds to the EpoR in the ER and promotes its cell surface expression. Thus, for the EpoR, Jak2 is not only essential for its signal transduction; it also acts as a chaperone along the biosynthetic pathway to regulate its surface expression (Huang et al. 2001). Replacement of all four prolines in the box-1 of the GHR by alanine residues resulted in the complete absence of both receptor and Jak2 phosphorylation. This modification, however, did not alter the rate and extent of receptor-bound growth hormone internalisation compared with a functional GHR, nor did it change its turnover and transport to the plasma membrane (Alves dos Santos et al. 2001). In addition, the receptor was still normally ubiquitinated and remained dependent on both an intact ubiquitin system and proteasome action for its internalisation. These experiments warrant the conclusion that, although endocytosis and degradation require the action of the ubiquitin system, they are fully independent of Jak2-dependent GHR signal transduction (Alves dos Santos et al. 2001). In addition, Jak2-*independent* GH signalling is probably not involved in trafficking, because binding of GH to its receptor does not effect GHR endocytosis and degradation (van Kerkhof et al. 2002).

GHR endocytosis is inhibited in the presence of proteasome inhibitors (van Kerkhof et al. 2000a). In addition, the downregulation of signal transduction as measured by the extent of tyrosine phosphorylation is inhibited by proteasome inhibitors. The obvious explanation would be that downregulation of GHR signal transduction is via endocytosis and lysosomal degradation. This appears not to be the case: The proteasome inhibitor MG132 prolongs the GH-induced activity of both GHR and Jak2 through inhibition of GHR and Jak2 tyrosine de-phosphorylation (Alves dos Santos et al. 2001). This result was confirmed when proteasome inhibitor was combined with ligand in an endocytosis-deficient GHR mutant. Thus proteasome action on tyrosine de-phosphorylation is independent of endocytosis. In addition, the proteasome plays a role in downregulation of GHR signal transduction.

Which mechanisms underlie the signal transduction downregulation of the GHR and JAK2 proteins? Experiments with a truncated tail mutant, GHR(1–369) revealed prolonged Jak2 phosphorylation caused by the loss of a phosphatase-binding site. In erythropoietin-induced cellular proliferation, recruitment of SHP-1 accomplishes dephosphorylation of Jak2 and subsequent termination of signal transduction (Jiao et al. 1996, Klingmuller et al. 1995). A similar role for SHP-1 in mediating the downregulation of Jak2 after stimulation of cells with GH has been proposed (Hackett et al. 1997). Our results with GHR(1–369) indicate that partial deletion of the C-terminal GHR tail leads to a prolonged Jak2 phosphorylation, presumably due to loss of a negative regulator binding site. This pattern of prolonged phosphorylation is similar to that of Jak2 in full wild-type GHRs treated with proteasome inhibitor. One explanation might be that the phosphatase activity is modulated by proteasome function, perhaps by degrading an inhibitory complex in a similar manner as for the inhibitor of the transcription factor NF-κBα (Yaron et al. 1997). This scenario suggests a stabilised phosphatase inhibitor complex in the presence of MG132 which prevents the de-phosphorylation of the JAK2 by SHP-1, thereby prolonging phosphorylation of both Jak2 and the GHR. In support of this model, SHP-1 degradation has been shown to be ubiquitin dependent in mast cells (Piao et al. 1996), suggesting that the proteasome is involved in SHP-1 regulation.

3.5
Signalling Control at the Endosomes

Signalling of tyrosine kinase receptors, like TrkA, EGF-R and the insulin receptor, continues after endocytosis (Ceresa et al. 1998; Grimes et al. 1996; Vieira et al. 1996). What happens to the signal transduction of the GHR after its internalisation? This question is relevant because the average time span of GH-GHR complexes at the cell surface is roughly the same as the transport time between endocytosis and segregation into the SE internal vesicles (5 min). The nature and intensity of signal transduction might be different because of different sets of signal transduction factors (Fig. 4). Co-immunoprecipitation of GH-GHR complexes before and after endocytosis showed that Jak2 as well as other activated proteins are bound to the GHR not only at the cell surface but also intracellularly, suggesting that the GHR signal transduction continues in endosomes (Alves dos Santos et al. 2001). Preliminary estimation of the tyrosine-phosphorylated proteins indicates that the nature of the signalling inside does not differ from signalling from the cell surface. Co-immunoprecipitation with anti-GH and immunoblotting with antibodies against the GH-binding domain also showed that both full-length and truncated forms of the GHR are present in endosomes, indicating that the receptor is indeed degraded from the cytosolic tail shortly after endocytosis. Together, these observations indicate that GHR signal transduction continues or resumes after endocytosis and that the signals, regenerated at the two cellular locations, do not differ substantially. Notably, binding of ligand to its cognate receptor may activate signal transduction pathways, which continue after internalisation, probably from endocytic vesicles and endosomes (Alves dos Santos et al. 2001; Vieira et al. 1996; Wiley and Burke 2001). Incorporation of receptors into internal endosomal vesicles segregates them from signalling molecules in the cytoplasm and provides an efficient way to terminate signalling.

4
The Potential of the System

GH is an important regulator of cellular metabolism and acts via the GHR. The expression level and the residence time at the cell surface together determine the number of GHRs at the surface. Unlike most known growth factor receptors, the GHR is synthesised and degraded continuously with a half-life of less than 60 min. Our research data indicate that, once synthesised, the number of receptors at the cell surface is mainly regulated by ubiquitin system-dependent uptake and degradation. This process is specific and, among growth factor receptors, unique for the GHR. Exogenous conditions, such as starvation and cell stress, stimulate GHR degradation. In addition, the uptake (and degradation) of GHRs is regulated by the ubiquitin system only if they are dimerised. Another significant area of GHR research concerns cell differentiation and regulation of metabolism. Model systems are the fibroblast cell lines 3T3-F442A and Ob-1771, which can be induced to differentiate into cells that possess the biochemical and morphological characteristics of adipocytes. One of many ways to exert anabolic activities has recently been illustrated in 3T3-F442A cells: GH, by activating ERKs, can modulate EGF-induced EGFR trafficking and signalling and initiates cross-talk between the GH and EGF signalling systems (Huang et al. 2003). When 3T3 cells become fully differentiated they are no longer able to proliferate and in the end apoptosis is inevitable, offering a model system to study metabolism and apoptosis. A second cell line, which expresses relatively high levels of endogenous GHRs, is IM-9 lymphoblasts. These human cells express several Epstein-Barr viral membrane proteins. Strikingly, in IM-9 cells GHR endocytosis depends on GH binding. Thus IM-9 cells are not only a natural system to study immune evasion mechanisms by Epstein-Barr virus, they will also facilitate study on the mechanism of GHR downregulation.

The merging the fields of cell biology and physiology will constitute a new interface for our insight in GHR function. Understanding the molecular principles of GHR trafficking as it is uniquely controlled by the ubiquitin-proteasome system will open up a new dimension in the understanding of how cells handle a multitude of signals to control cell differentiation, stress, apoptosis and anabolic and catabolic pathways.

Acknowledgements The authors thank Marcel Roza, Toine ten Broeke, Rachel Leckie, Aaron Ciechanover, Alan Schwartz, Guojun Bu, Judith Klumperman, Erica Vallon and Monique van den Eijnden for their help, contributions and support. This work on the GHR was mainly financed by the UMC Utrecht and by grants of the Netherlands Organization for Scientific Research (NWO-902-23-192) and the European Union (ERBFMRXCT96-0026).

References

Aberle H, Bauer A, Stappert J, Kispert A, Kemler R (1997 β-Catenin is a target for the ubiquitin-proteasome pathway. EMBO J 16:3797–3804

Adams TE, Hansen JA, Starr R, Nicola NA, Hilton DJ, Billestrup N (1998) Growth hormone preferentially induces the rapid, transient expression of SOCS-3, a novel inhibitor of cytokine receptor signaling. J Biol Chem 273:1285–1287

Alves dos Santos CM, ten Broeke T, Strous GJ (2001) Growth hormone receptor ubiquitination, endocytosis, and degradation are independent of signal transduction via Janus kinase 2. J Biol Chem 276:32635–32641

Alves dos Santos CM, van Kerkhof P, Strous GJ (2001) The signal transduction of the growth hormone receptor is regulated by the ubiquitin/proteasome system and continues after endocytosis. J Biol Chem 276:10839–10846

Argetsinger LS, Campbell GS, Yang XN, Witthuhn BA, Silvennoinen O, Ihle JN, Carter Su C (1993) Identification of JAK2 as a growth hormone receptor-associated tyrosine kinase. Cell 74:237–244

Argetsinger LS, Hsu GW, Myers MG, Billestrup N, White MF, Carter Su C (1995) Growth hormone, interferon-gamma, and leukemia inhibitory factor promoted tyrosyl phosphorylation of insulin receptor substrate-1. J Biol Chem 270:14685–14692

Argetsinger LS, Carter Su C (1996) Mechanism of signaling by growth hormone receptor. Physiol Rev 76:1089–1107

Ayling RM, Ross RJM, Towner P, Vonlaue S, Finidori J, Moutoussamy S, Buchanan CR, Clayton PE, Norman MR (1999) New growth hormone receptor exon 9 mutation causes genetic short stature. Acta Paediatrica 88:168–172

Ayoub MA, Couturier C, Lucas-Meunier E, Angers S, Fossier P, Bouvier M, Jockers R (2002) Monitoring of ligand-independent dimerization and ligand-induced conformational changes of melatonin receptors in living cells by bioluminescence resonance energy transfer. J Biol Chem 277:21522–21528

Bazan JF (1990) Structural design and molecular evolution of a cytokine receptor superfamily. Proc Natl Acad Sci USA 87:6934–6938

Billestrup N, Bouchelouche P, Allevato G, Ilondo M, Nielsen JH (1995) Growth hormone receptor C-terminal domains required for growth hormone-induced intracellular free Ca^{2+} oscillations and gene transcription. Proc Natl Acad Sci USA 92:2725–2729

Boll W, Rapoport I, Brunner C, Modis Y, Prehn S, Kirchhausen T (2002) The mu2 subunit of the clathrin adaptor AP-2 binds to FDNPVY and YppO sorting signals at distinct sites. Traffic 3:590–600

Bonifacino JS, Traub LM (2003) Signals for sorting of transmembrane proteins to endosomes and lysosomes. Annu Rev Biochem (in press)

Campbell GS, Meyer DJ, Raz R, Levy DE, Schwartz J, Carter-Su C (1995) Activation of acute phase response factor (APRF)/Stat3 transcription factor by growth hormone. J Biol Chem 270:3974–3979

Carter-Su C, King AP, Argetsinger LS, Smit LS, Vanderkuur J, Campbell GS (1996) Signalling pathway of GH. Endocr J 43:S65–70

Carter-Su C, Schwartz J, Smit LS (1996) Molecular mechanism of growth hormone action. Annu Rev Physiol 58:187–207

Casanueva FF (1992) Physiology of growth hormone secretion and action. Endcrinol Metab Clin North Am 21:483–517

Ceresa BP, Kao AW, Santeler SR, Pessin JE (1998) Inhibition of clathrin-mediated endocytosis selectively attenuates specific insulin receptor signal transduction pathways. Mol Cell Biol 18:3862–3870

Cheatham B, Vlahos CJ, Cheatham L, Wang L, Blenis J, Kahn CR (1994) Phosphatidylinositol 3-kinase activation is required for insulin stimulation of pp70 S6 kinase, DNA synthesis, and glucose transporter translocation. Mol Cell Biol 14:4902–4911

Chen C, Brinkworth R, Waters MJ (1997) The role of receptor dimerization domain residues in growth hormone signaling. J Biol Chem 272:5133–140

Chen W-J, Goldstein JL, Brown MS (1990) NPXY, a sequence often found in cytoplasmic tails, is required for coated pit-mediated internalization of the low density lipoprotein receptor. J Biol Chem 265:3116–3123

Chen WY, Wight DC, Wagner TE, Kopchick JJ (1990) Expression of a mutated bovine growth hormone gene suppresses growth of transgenic mice. Proc Natl Acad Sci USA 87:5061–5065

Chen ZJ, Hagler J, Palombella VJ, Melandri F, Scherer D, Ballard D, Maniatis T (1995) Signal-induced site-specific phosphorylation targets I(kappa)Balpha to the ubiquitin-proteasome pathway. Gene Dev 9:1586–1597

Cobb MH, Goldsmith EJ (1995) How MAP kinases are regulated. J Biol Chem 270:14843–14846

Collawn JF, Stangel M, Kuhn LA, Esekogwu V, Jing SQ, Trowbridge IS, Tainer JA (1990) Transferrin receptor internalization sequence yxrf implicates a tight turn as the structural recognition motif for endocytosis. Cell 63:1061–1072

Constantinescu SN, Keren T, Socolovsky M, Nam Hs H, Henis YI, Lodish HF (2001) Ligand-independent oligomerization of cell-surface erythropoietin receptor is mediated by the transmembrane domain. Proc Natl Acad Sci USA 98:4379–4384

Craiu A, Gaczynska M, Akopian T, Gramm CF, Fenteany G, Goldberg AL, Rock KL (1997) Lactacystin and clasto-lactacystin beta-lactone modify multiple proteasome beta-subunits and inhibit intracellular protein degradation and major histocompatibility complex class I antigen presentation. J Biol Chem 272:13437–13445

Cunningham BC, Ultsch M, De Vos AM, Mulkerrin MG, Clauser KR, Wells JA (1991) Dimerization of the extracellular domain of the human growth hormone receptor by a single hormone molecule. Science 254:821–825

Darnell JE, Jr. (1997) STATs and gene regulation. Science 277:1630–1635

Dastot F, Sobrier ML, Duquesnoy P, Duriez B, Goossens M, Amselem S (1996) Alternatively spliced forms in the cytoplasmic domain of the human growth hormone (GH) receptor regulate its ability to generate a soluble GH-binding protein. Proc Natl Acad Sci USA 93:10723–10728

Dautry-Varsat A, Ciechanover A, Lodish HF (1983) pH and the recycling of transferrin during receptor-mediated endocytosis. Proc Natl Acad Sci USA 80:2258–2262

Davis RJ (1993) The mitogen-activated protein kinase signal transduction pathway. J Biol Chem 268:14553–14556

De Craene JO, Soetens O, Andre B (2001) The Npr1 kinase controls biosynthetic and endocytic sorting of the yeast Gap1 permease. J Biol Chem 276: 43939–43948

de Vos AM, Ultsch M, Kossiakoff AA (1992) Human growth hormone and extracellular domain of its receptor: crystal structure of the complex. Science 255:306–312

Frank SJ (2001) Growth hormone signalling and its regulation: Preventing too much of a good thing. Growth Horm IGF Res 11:201–212

Fuh G, Cunningham BC, Fukunaga R, Nagata S, Goeddel DV, Wells JA (1992) Rational design of potent antagonists to the growth hormone receptor. Science 256:1677–1680

Galan JM, Moreau V, Andre B, Volland C, Haguenauer-Tsapis R (1996) Ubiquitination mediated by the npi1p/rsp5p ubiquitin-protein ligase is required for endocytosis of the yeast uracil permease. J Biol Chem 271:10946–10952

Galan JM, Haguenauer-Tsapis R (1997) Ubiquitin Lys63 is involved in ubiquitination of a yeast plasma membrane protein. EMBO J 16:5847–5854

Gallusser A, Kirchhausen T (1993) The beta 1 and beta 2 subunits of the AP complexes are the clathrin coat assembly components. EMBO J 12:5237–5244

Gaur S, Yamaguchi H, Goodman HM (1996a) Growth hormone regulates cytosolic free Ca^{2+} in rat fat cells by maintaining L-type calcium channels. Am J Physiol Cell Physiol 270:C1478–C1484

Gaur S, Yamaguchi H, Goodman HM (1996b) Growth hormone increases Ca^{2+} uptake in rat fat cells by a mechanism dependent on protein kinase C. Am J Physiol Cell Physiol 270:C1485–C1492

Gebert CA, Park SH, Waxman DJ (1999) Termination of growth hormone pulse-induced STAT5b signaling. Mol Endocrinol 13:38–56

Gent J, van Kerkhof P, Roza M, Bu G, Strous GJ (2002) Ligand-independent growth hormone receptor dimerization occurs in the endoplasmic reticulum and is required for ubiquitin system-dependent endocytosis. Proc Natl Acad Sci USA 99:9858–9863

Gent J, Van Den Eijnden M, Van Kerkhof P, Strous GJ (2003) Dimerization and signal transduction of the GH receptor. Mol Endocrinol (in press)

Geuze HJ, Slot JW, Strous GJ, Lodish HF, Schwartz AL (1983) Intracellular site of asialoglycoprotein receptor-ligand uncoupling: Double-label immunoelectron microscopy during receptor-mediated endocytosis. Cell 32:277–287

Geuze HJ (1998) The role of endosomes and lysosomes in MHC class II functioning. Immunology Today 19:282–287

Glickman JA, Conibear E, Pearse BMF (1989) Specificity of binding of clathrin adaptors to signals on the mannose-6-phosphate/insulin-like growth factor II receptor. EMBO J 8:1041–1047

Godowski PJ, Leung DW, Meacham LR, Galgani JP, Hellmiss R, Keret R, Rotwein P, Wood WI (1989) Charaterization of the human growth hormone receptor gene and demonstration of a partial gene deletion in two patients with Laron-type dwarfism. Proc Natl Acad Sci USA 86:8083–8087

Goodman OB, Krupnick JG, Santini F, Gurevich VV, Penn RB, Gagnon AW, Keen J, Benovic JL (1996) Beta-arrestin acts as a clathrin adaptor in endocytosis of the beta-2-adrenergic receptor. Nature 383:447–450

Govers R, van Kerkhof P, Schwartz AL, Strous GJ (1997) Linkage of the ubiquitin-conjugating system and the endocytic pathway in ligand-induced internalization of the growth hormone receptor. EMBO J 16:4851–4858

Govers R, van Kerkhof P, Schwartz AL, Strous GJ (1998) Di-leucine-mediated internalization of ligand by a truncated growth hormone receptor is independent of the ubiquitin conjugation system. J Biol Chem 273:16426–16433

Govers R, ten Broeke T, van Kerkhof P, Schwartz AL, Strous GJ (1999) Identification of a novel ubiquitin conjugation motif, required for ligand-induced internalization of the growth hormone receptor. EMBO J 18:28–36

Grimes ML, Zhou J, Beattie EC, Yuen EC, Hall DE, Valletta JS, Topp KS, LaVail JH, Bunnett NW, Mobley WC (1996) Endocytosis of activated trkA: evidence that nerve growth factor induces formation of signaling endosomes. J Neurosci 16:7950–7964

Gu F, Aniento F, Parton RG, Gruenberg J (1997) Functional dissection of COP-I subunits in the biogenesis of multivesicular endosomes. J Cell Biol 139:1183–1195

Hackett RH, Wang YD, Sweitzer S, Feldman G, Wood WI, Larner AC (1997) Mapping of a cytoplasmic domain of the human growth hormone receptor that regulates rates of inactivation of jak2 and stat proteins. J Biol Chem 272:11128–11132

Harding PA, Wang X, Okada S, Chen WY, Wan W, Kopchick JJ (1996) Growth hormone (GH) and a GH antagonist promote GH receptor dimerization and internalization. J Biol Chem 271:6708–6712

Helliwell SB, Losko S, Kaiser CA (2001) Components of a ubiquitin ligase complex specify polyubiquitination and intracellular trafficking of the general amino acid permease. J Cell Biol 153:649–62

Hershko A, Ciechanover A (1998) The ubiquitin system. Annu Rev Biochem 67:425–479

Hicke L, Zanolari B, Riezman H (1998) Cytoplasmic tail phosphorylation of the alpha-factor receptor is required for its ubiquitination and internalization. J Cell Biol 141:349–358

Hicke L (2001) Protein regulation by monoubiquitin. Nat Rev Mol Cell Biol 2:195–201

Holtzman E, Dominitz R (1968) Cytochemical studies of lysosomes, golgi apparatus and endoplasmic reticulum in secretion and protein uptake by adrenal medulla cells of the rat. J Histochem Cytochem 16:320–336

Hopkins CR, Gibson A, Shipman M, Miller K (1990) Movement of internalized ligand-receptor complexes along a continuous endosomal reticulum. Nature 346:335–339

Huang KM, D'Hondt K, Riezman H, Lemmon SK (1999) Clathrin functions in the absence of heterotetrameric adaptors and AP180-related proteins in yeast. EMBO J 18:3897–3908

Huang LJ, Constantinescu SN, Lodish HF (2001) The N-terminal domain of janus kinase 2 is required for Golgi processing and cell surface expression of erythropoietin receptor. Mol Cell 8:1327–1338

Huang Y, Kim SO, Jiang J, Frank SJ (2003) Growth hormone-induced phosphorylation of epidermal growth factor (EGF) receptor in 3T3-F442A cells: Modulation of EGF-induced trafficking and signalling. J Biol Chem 278:18902–18913

Iida K, Takahashi Y, Kaji H, Takahashi MO, Okimura Y, Nose O, Abe H, Chihara K (1999) Functional characterization of truncated growth hormone (GH) receptor-(1–277) causing partial GH insensitivity syndrome with high GH-binding protein. J Clin Endocrinol Metabol 84:1011–1016

Ilondo MM, Courtoy PJ, Geiger D, Carpentier J, Rousseau GG, de Meyts P (1986) Intracellular potassium depletion in IM-9 lymphocytes suppresses the slowly dissociating component of human growth hormone binding and the down-regulation of its receptors but does not affect insulin receptors. Proc Natl Acad Sci USA 83:6460–6464

Isaksson OG, Eden S, Jansson JO (1985) Mode of action of pituitary growth hormone on target cells. Annu Rev Physiol 47:483–499

Jansson JO, Albertsson-Wikland K, Eden S, Thorngren KG, Isaksson O (1982) Effect of frequency of growth hormone administration on longitudinal bone growth and body weight in hypophysectomized rats. Acta Physiol Scand 114:261–265

Jeffers M, Taylor GA, Weidner KM, Omura S, Vandewoude GF (1997) Degradation of the met tyrosine kinase receptor by the ubiquitin-proteasome pathway. Mol Cell Biol 17:799–808

Jiao H, Berrada, Yang W, Tabrizi M, Platanias LC, Yi T (1996) Direct association with and dephosphorylation of JAK2 kinase by the SH2-domain-containing protein tyrosine phosphatase SHP-1. Mol Cell Biol 16:6985–6992

Joazeiro CA, Wing SS, Huang H, Leverson JD, Hunter T, Liu YC (1999) The tyrosine kinase negative regulator c-Cbl as a RING-type, E2-dependent ubiquitin-protein ligase. Science 286:309–312

Johnson LS, Dunn KW, Pytowski B, Mcgraw TE (1993) Endosome acidification and receptor trafficking—bafilomycin a(1) slows receptor externalization by a mechanism involving the receptors internalization motif. Mol Biol Cell 4:1251–1266

Kirchhausen T (1999) Adaptors for clathrin-mediated traffic. Annu Rev Cell Dev Biol 15:705–732

Klapisz E, Sorokina I, Lemeer S, Pijnenburg M, Verkleij AJ, Van Bergen En Henegouwen PM (2002) A ubiquitin-interacting motif (UIM) is essential for Eps15 and Eps15R ubiquitination. J Biol Chem 277:30746–30753

Klausner RD, Ashwell G, van Renswoude J, Harford JB, Bridges KR (1983) Binding of apotransferrin to K562 cells: Explanation of the transferrin cycle. Proc Natl Acad Sci USA 80:2263–2266

Kleijmeer MJ, Morkowski S, Griffith JM, Rudensky AY, Geuze HJ (1997) Major histo-compatibility complex class II compartments in human and mouse B lym-phoblasts represent conventional endocytic compartments. J Cell Biol 139:639–649

Klingmuller U, Lorenz U, Cantley LC, Neel BG, Lodish HF (1995) Specific recruit-ment of SH-PTP1 to the erythropoietin receptor causes inactivation of jak2 and termination of proliferative signals. Cell 80:729–738

Kölling R, Hollenberg CP (1994) The ABC-transporter Ste6 accumulates in the plas-ma membrane in a ubiquitinated form in endocytosis mutants. EMBO J 13:3261–3271

Krebs DL, Hilton DJ (2000) SOCS: Physiological suppressors of cytokine signaling. J Cell Science 113:2813–2819

Krupnick JG, Goodman OB, Keen JH, Benovic JL (1997) Arrestin/clathrin interac-tion—Localization of the clathrin binding domain of nonvisual arrestins to the carboxyl terminus. J Biol Chem 272:15011–15016

Laporte SA, Oakley RH, Zhang J, Holt JA, Ferguson SSG, Caron MG, Barak LS (1999) The beta(2)-adrenergic receptor/beta-arrestin complex recruits the clathrin adaptor AP-2 during endocytosis. Proc Natl Acad Sci USA 96:3712–3717

Laporte SA, Oakley RH, Holt JA, Barak LS, Caron MG (2000) The interaction of beta-arrestin with the AP-2 adaptor is required for the clustering of beta(2)-ad-renergic receptor into clathrin-coated pits. J Biol Chem 275:23120–23126

Laron Z, Pertzelan A, Mannheimer S (1966) Genetic pituitary dwarfism with high se-rum concentration of growth hormone–a new inborn error of metabolism? Isr J Med Sci 2:152–155

Lee PSW, Wang Y, Dominguez MG, Yeung YG, Murphy MA, Bowtell DDL, Stanley ER (1999) The Cbl protooncoprotein stimulates CSF-1 receptor multiubiquitination and endocytosis, and attenuates macrophage proliferation. EMBO J 18:3616–3628

Levkowitz G, Waterman H, Zamir E, Kam Z, Oved S, Langdon WY, Beguinot L, Geiger B, Yarden Y (1998) c-Cbl/Sli-1 regulates endocytic sorting and ubiquitina-tion of the epidermal growth factor receptor. Genes Dev 12:3663–3674

Levkowitz G, Waterman H, Ettenberg SA, Katz M, Tsygankov AY, Alroy I, Lavi S, Iwai K, Reiss Y, Ciechanover A, Lipkowitz S, Yarden Y (1999) Ubiquitin ligase activity and tyrosine phosphorylation underlie suppression of growth factor signaling by c-Cbl/Sli-1. Mol Cell 4:1029–1040

Maamra M, Finidori J, Vonlaue S, Simon S, Justice S, Webster J, Dower S, Ross R (1999) Studies with a growth hormone antagonist and dual-fluorescent confocal microscopy demonstrate that the full-length human growth hormone receptor, but not the truncated isoform, is very rapidly internalized independent of Jak2-Stat5 signaling. J Biol Chem 274:14791–14798

Marks MS, Ohno H, Kirchhausen T, Bonifacino SJ (1997) Protein sorting by tyrosine-based signals: Adapting to the Ys and wherefores. Trends Cell Biol 7:124–128

Martinez-Moczygemba M, Huston DP (2001) Proteasomal regulation of betac signaling reveals a novel mechanism for cytokine receptor heterotypic desensitization. J Clin Invest 108:1797–1806

Martin-Fernandez M, Clarke DT, Tobin MJ, Jones SV, Jones GR (2002) Preformed oligomeric epidermal growth factor receptors undergo an ectodomain structure change during signaling. Biophys J 82:2415–2427

Matsumoto A, Masuhara M, Mitsui K, Yokouchi M, Ohtsubo M, Misawa H, Miyajima A, Yoshimura A (1997) CIS, a cytokine inducible SH2 protein, is a target of the JAK-STAT5 pathway and modulates STAT5 activation. Blood 89:3148–3154

Matsumoto A, Seki Y, Kubo M, Ohtsuka S, Suzuki A, Hayashi I, Tsuji K, Nakahata T, Okabe M, Yamada S, Yoshimura A (1999) Suppression of STAT5 functions in liver, mammary glands, and T cells in cytokine-inducible SH2-containing protein 1 transgenic mice. Mol Cell Biol 19:6396–6407

Mellado M, Rodriguez-Frade JM, Kremer L, von Kobbe C, de Ana AM, Merida I, Martinez AC (1997) Conformational changes required in the human growth hormone receptor for growth hormone signaling. J Biol Chem 272:9189–9196

Metcalf D, Greenhalgh CJ, Viney E, Willson TA, Starr R, Nicola NA, Hilton DJ, Alexander WS (2000) Gigantism in mice lacking suppressor of cytokine signalling-2. Nature 405:1069–1073

Miller JD, Tannenbaum GS, Colle E, Guyda HJ (1982) Daytime pulsatile growth hormone secretion during childhood and adolescence. J Clin Endocrinol Metab 55:989–994

Miyake S, Lupher ML, Druker B, Band H (1998) The tyrosine kinase regulator Cbl enhances the ubiquitination and degradation of the platelet-derived growth factor receptor alpha. Proc Natl Acad Sci USA 95:7927–7932

Mori S, Tanaka K, Omura S, Saito Y (1995) Degradation process of ligand-stimulated platelet-derived growth factor beta-receptor involves ubiquitin-proteasome proteolytic pathway. J Biol Chem 270:29447–29452

Moriki T, Maruyama H, Maruyama IN (2001) Activation of preformed EGF receptor dimers by ligand-induced rotation of the transmembrane domain. J Mol Biol 311:1011–1026

Moutoussamy S, Kelly PA, Finidori J (1998) Growth-hormone-receptor and cytokine-receptor-family signaling. Eur J Biochem 255:1–11

Murphy LJ, Lazarus L (1984) The mouse fibroblast growth hormone receptor: Ligand processing and receptor modulation and turnover. Endocrinology 115:1625–1632

Ohno H, Stewart J, Fournier MC, Bosshart H, Rhee I, Miyatake S, Saito T, Gallusser A, Kirchhausen T, Bonifacino JS (1995) Interaction of tyrosine-based sorting signals with clathrin-associated proteins. Science 269:1872–1875

Petrelli A, Gilestro GF, Lanzardo S, Comoglio PM, Migone N, Giordano S (2002) The endophilin-CIN85-Cbl complex mediates ligand-dependent down-regulation of c-Met. Nature 416:187–190

Piao XH, Paulson R, Vandergeer P, Pawson T, Bernstein A (1996) Oncogenic mutation in the kit receptor tyrosine kinase alters substrate specificity and induces
degradation of the protein tyrosine phosphatase shp-1. Proc Natl Acad Sci USA
93:14665–14669

Piguet V, Gu F, Foti M, Demaurex N, Gruenberg J, Carpentier JL, Trono D (1999)
Nef-induced CD4 degradation: A diacidic-based motif in Nef functions as a lysosomal targeting signal through the binding of beta-COP in endosomes. Cell
97:63–73

Pircher TJ, Petersen H, Gustafsson JA, Haldosen LA (1999) Extracellular signal-regulated kinase (ERK) interacts with signal transducer and activator of transcription
(STAT) 5a. Mol Endocrinol 13:555–565

Plemper RK, Wolf DH (1999) Retrograde protein translocation: ERADication of secretory proteins in health and disease. Tr Biochem Sci 24:266–270

Polo S, Sigismund S, Faretta M, Guidi M, Capua MR, Bossi G, Chen H, De Camilli P,
Di Fiore PP (2002) A single motif responsible for ubiquitin recognition and
monoubiquitination in endocytic proteins. Nature 416:451–455

Raiborg C, Bache KG, Gillooly DJ, Madshus IH, Stang E, Stenmark H (2002) Hrs
sorts ubiquitinated proteins into clathrin-coated microdomains of early endosomes. Nat Cell Biol 4:394–398

Ram PA, Waxman DJ (1999) SOCS/CIS protein inhibition of growth hormone-stimu-
lated STAT5 signaling by multiple mechanisms. J Biol Chem 274:35553–35561

Rapoport I, Chen YC, Cupers P, Shoelson SE, Kirchhausen T 1998 Dileucine-based
sorting signals bind to the beta chain of AP-1 at a site distinct and regulated differently from the tyrosine-based motif-binding site EMBO J 17:2148–2155

Raposo G, Tenza D, Murphy DM, Berson JF, Marks MS (2001) Distinct protein sorting and localization to premelanosomes, melanosomes, and lysosomes in pig-
mented melanocytic cells. J Cell Biol 152:809–824

Remy I, Wilson IA, Michnick SW (1999) Erythropoietin receptor activation by a ligand-induced conformation change. Science 283:990–993

Ridderstrale M, Tornqvist H (1994) PI-3-kinase inhibitor Wortmannin blocks the insulin-like effects of growth hormone in isolated rat adipocytes. Biochem Biophys
Res Commun 203:306–310

Rocca A, Lamaze C, Subtil A, Dautry-Varsat A (2001) Involvement of the ubiquitin/
proteasome system in sorting of the interleukin 2 receptor beta chain to late endocytic compartments. Mol Biol Cell 12:1293–1301

Rosenbloom AL (2000) Physiology and disorders of the growth hormone receptor
(GHR) and GH-GHR signal transduction. Endocrine 12:107–119

Ross RJ, Esposito N, Shen XY, Von Laue S, Chew SL, Dobson PR, Finidori J (1997) A
short isoform of the human growth hormone receptor functions as a dominant
negative inhibitor of the full-length receptor and generates large amounts of
binding protein. Mol Endocrinol 11:265–273

Ross RJM (1999) The GH receptor and GH insensitivity. Growth Horm IGF Res
9:42–45

Roth AF, Davis NG (2000) Ubiquitination of the PEST-like endocytosis signal of the
yeast α-factor receptor. J Biol Chem 275:8143–8153

Rui L, Carter-Su C (1999) Identification of SH2-B as a potent cytoplasmic activator
of the tyrosine kinase Janus kinase 2. Proc Natl Acad Sci USA 96:7172–7177

Sachse M, van Kerkhof P, Strous GJ, Klumperman J (2001) The ubiquitin-dependent endocytosis motif is required for efficient incorporation of growth hormone receptor in clathrin-coated pits, but not clathrin-coated lattices. J Cell Sci 114:3943–3952

Sachse M, Urbe S, Oorschot V, Strous GJ, Klumperman J (2002) Bilayered clathrin coats on endosomal vacuoles are involved in protein sorting toward lysosomes. Mol Biol Cell 13:1313–1328

Sachse M, Strous GJ, Klumperman J (2003) The AAA-type ATPase hVPS4 regulates association of bilayered clathrin coats on endosomal vacuoles. In preparation

Saito Y, Teshima R, Yamazaki T, Ikebuchi H, Sawada JC (1994) Ligand-induced internalization and phosphorylation-dependent degradation of growth hormone receptor in human IM-9 cells. Mol Cell Endocrinol 106:67–74

Santini F, Gaidarov I, Keen JH (2002) G protein-coupled receptor/arrestin3 modulation of the endocytic machinery. J Cell Biol 156:665–676

Schantl JA, Roza M, de Jong AP, Strous GJ (2003) Small glutamine-rich tetratricopeptide repeat-containing protein interacts with the ubiquitin-dependent endocytosis motif of the growth hormone receptor. Biochem J (in press)

Schmid S, Fuchs R, Kielian M, Helenius A, Mellman I (1989) Acidification of endosome subpopulations in wild-type Chinese hamster ovary cells and temperature-sensitive acidification-defective mutants. J Cell Biol 108:1291–300

Schmid SL, Fuchs R, Male P, Mellman I (1988) Two distinct subpopulations of endosomes involved in membrane recycling and transport to lysosomes. Cell 52:73–83

Shenoy SK, McDonald PH, Kohout TA, Lefkowitz RJ (2001) Regulation of receptor fate by ubiquitination of activated β2-adrenergic receptor and β-arrestin. Science 294:1307–1313

Shih SC, Slopermould KE, Hicke L (2000) Monoubiquitin carries a novel internalization signal that is appended to activated receptors. EMBO J 19:187–198

Shih SC, Katzmann DJ, Schnell JD, Sutanto M, Emr SD, Hicke L (2002) Epsins and Vps27p/Hrs contain ubiquitin-binding domains that function in receptor endocytosis. Nat Cell Biol 4:389–393

Shin J, Dunbrack RL, Lee JS, Strominger JL (1991) Phosphorylation-dependent down-modulation of CD4 requires a specific structure within the cytoplasmic domain of CD4. J Biol Chem 266:10658–10665

Soetens O, De Craene JO, Andre B (2001) Ubiquitin is required for sorting to the vacuole of the yeast Gap1 permease. J Biol Chem 276:43949–43957

Sorkin A, Carpenter G (1993) Interaction of activated EGF receptors with coated pit adaptins. Science 261:612–615

Sorkin A, Waters CM (1993) Endocytosis of growth factor receptors. Bioessays 15:375–382

Sorkin A, Mazzotti M, Sorkina T, Scotto L, Beguinot L (1996) Epidermal growth factor receptor interaction with clathrin adaptors is mediated by the Tyr(974)-containing internalization motif. J Biol Chem 271:13377–13384

Sotiropoulos A, Perrot Applanat M, Dinerstein H, Pallier A, Postel Vinay MC, Finidori J, Kelly PA (1994) Distinct cytoplasmic regions of the growth hormone receptor are required for activation of JAK2, mitogen-activated protein kinase, and transcription. Endocrinology 135:1292–1298

Soubeyran P, Kowanetz K, Szymkiewicz I, Langdon WY, Dikic I (2002) Cbl-CIN85-endophilin complex mediates ligand-induced down-regulation of EGF receptors. Nature 416:183–187

Souza SC, Frick GP, Yip R, Lobo RB, Tai L, Goodman HM (1994) Growth hormone stimulates tyrosine phosphorylation of insulin receptor substrate-1. J Biol Chem 269:30085–30088

Starr R, Willson TA, Niney EM, Murray LJL, Rayner JR, Jenkins BJ, Gonda TJ (1997) A family of cytokine-inducible inhibitors of signaling. Nature 387:917–921

Staub O, Gautschi I, Ishikawa T, Breitschopf K, Ciechanover A, Schild L, Rotin D (1997) Regulation of stability and function of the epithelial Na$^+$ channel (ENaC) by ubiquitination. EMBO J 16:6325–6336

Stofega MR, Wang H, Ullrich A, Carter-Su C (1998) Growth hormone regulation of SIRP and SHP-2 tyrosyl phosphorylation and association. J Biol Chem 273:7112–7117

Stofega MR, Argetsinger LS, Wang H, Ullrich A, Carter-Su C (2000) Negative regulation of growth hormone receptor/JAK2 signaling by signal regulatory protein alpha. J Biol Chem 275:28222–8229

Stofega MR, Herrington J, Billestrup N, Carter-Su C (2000) Mutation of the SHP-2 binding site in growth hormone (GH) receptor prolongs GH-promoted tyrosyl phosphorylation of GH receptor, JAK2, and STAT5B. Mol Endocrinol 14:1338–1350

Strous G, Gent J (2002) Dimerization, ubiquitylation and endocytosis go together in growth hormone receptor function. FEBS Lett 529:102–109

Strous GJ, van Kerkhof P, Govers R, Ciechanover A, Schwartz AL (1996) The ubiquitin conjugation system is required for ligand-induced endocytosis and degradation of the growth hormone receptor. EMBO J 15:3806–3812

Strous GJ, Govers R (1999) The ubiquitin-proteasome system and endocytosis. J Cell Sci 112:1417–1423

Strous GJ, van Kerkhof P (2002) The ubiquitin-proteasome pathway and the regulation of growth hormone receptor availability. Mol Cell Endocrinol 197:143–151

Swaminathan S, Amerik AY, Hochstrasser M (1999) The Doa4 deubiquitinating enzyme is required for ubiquitin homeostasis in yeast. Mol Biol Cell 10:2583–2594

Terhaar E, Harrison SC, Kirchhausen T (2000) Peptide-in-groove interactions link target proteins to the beta-propeller of clathrin. Proc Natl Acad Sci USA 97:1096–1100

Terrell J, Shih S, Dunn R, Hicke L (1998) A function for monoubiquitination in the internalization of a G protein-coupled receptor. Mol Cell 1:193–202

Thrower JS, Hoffman L, Rechsteiner M, Pickart CM (2000) Recognition of the polyubiquitin proteolytic signal. EMBO J 19:94–102

Tollet-Egnell P, Floresmorales A, Stavreusevers A, Sahlin L, Norstedt G (1999) Growth hormone regulation of SOCS-2, SOCS-3, and CIS messenger ribonucleic acid expression in the rat. Endocrinology 140:3693–3704

Trainer PJ, Drake WM, Katznelson L, Freda PU, Herman-Bonert V, van der Lely AJ, Dimaraki EV, Stewart PM, Friend KE, Vance ML, Besser GM, Scarlett JA, Thorner MO, Parkinson C, Klibanski A, Powell JS, Barkan AL, Sheppard MC, Malsonado M, Rose DR, Clemmons DR, Johannsson G, Bengtsson BA, Stavrou S, Kleinberg DL, Cook DM, Phillips LS, Bidlingmaier M, Strasburger CJ, Hackett S, Zib K,

Bennett WF, Davis RJ (2000) Treatment of acromegaly with the growth hormone-receptor antagonist pegvisomant. N Engl J Med 342:1171–1177

Ungureanu D, Saharinen P, Junttila I, Hilton DJ, Silvennoinen O (2002) Regulation of Jak2 through the ubiquitin-proteasome pathway involves phosphorylation of Jak2 on Y1007 and interaction with SOCS-1. Mol Cell Biol 22:3316–3326

Urbé S, Mills IG, Stenmark H, Kitamura N, Clague MJ (2000) Endosomal localization and receptor dynamics determine tyrosine phosphorylation of hepatocyte growth factor-regulated tyrosine kinase substrate. Mol Cell Biol 20:7685–7692

Urbé S, Sachse M, Preisinger C, Barr FA, Strous GJ, Klumperman J, Clague MJ (2003) The UIM domain of Hrs is required for EGF-dependent phosphorylation and prevents entry to lumenal vesicles. J Cell Sci (in press)

van Delft S, Govers R, Strous GJ, Verkleij AJ, van Bergen en Henegouwen PM (1997) Epidermal growth factor induces ubiquitination of Eps15. J Biol Chem 272:14013–14016

van Kerkhof P, Govers R, Alves dosSantos CMA, Strous GJ (2000a) Endocytosis and degradation of the growth hormone receptor are proteasome-dependent. J Biol Chem 275:1575–1580

van Kerkhof P, Sachse M, Klumperman J, Strous GJ (2000b) Growth hormone receptor ubiquitination coincides with recruitment to clathrin-coated membrane domains. J Biol Chem 276:3778–3784

van Kerkhof P, Alves dos Santos CM, Sachse M, Klumperman J, Bu G, Strous GJ (2001) Proteasome inhibitors block a late step in lysosomal transport of selected membrane but not soluble proteins. Mol Biol Cell 12:2556–2566

van Kerkhof P, Strous GJ (2001) The ubiquitin-proteasome pathway regulates lysosomal degradation of the growth hormone receptor and its ligand. Biochem Soc Trans 29:488–493

van Kerkhof P, Smeets M, Strous GJ (2002) The Ubiquitin-proteasome pathway regulates the availability of the GH receptor. Endocrinology 143:1243–1252

van Kerkhof P, Vallon E, Strous GJ (2003) A method to increase the number of growth hormone receptors at the surface of cells. Mol Cell Endocrinol 201:57–62

VanderKuur J, Allevato G, Billestrup N, Norstedt G, Carter-Su C (1995) Growth hormone-promoted tyrosyl phosphorylation of SHC proteins and SHC association with Grb2. J Biol Chem 270:7587–7593

VanderKuur JA, Wang X, Zhang L, Campbell GS, Allevato G, Bellestrup N, Norstedt G, Carter-Su C (1994) Domains of the growth hormone receptor required for association and activation of JAK2 tyrosine kinase. J Biol Chem 269:21709–21717

VanderKuur JA, Butch ER, Waters SB, Pessin JE, Guan KL, CarterSu C (1997) Signaling molecules involved in coupling growth hormone receptor to mitogen-activated protein kinase activation. Endocrinology 138:4301–4307

Verdier F, Walrafen P, Hubert N, Chretien S, Gisselbrecht S, Lacombe C, Mayeux P (2000) Proteasomes regulate the duration of erythropoietin receptor activation by controlling down-regulation of cell surface receptors. J Biol Chem 275:18375–18381

Vieira AV, Lamaze C, Schmid SL (1996) Control of EGF receptor signaling by clathrin-mediated endocytosis. Science 274:2086–2089

Vleurick L, Pezet A, Kuhn ER, Decuypere E, Edery M (1999) A beta-turn endocytic code is required for optimal internalization of the growth hormone receptor but not for alpha-adaptin association. Mol Endocrinol 13:1823–1831

Wang X, Darus CJ, Xu BC, Kopchick JJ (1996) Identification of growth hormone receptor (GHR) tyrosine residues required for GHR phosphorylation and JAK2 and STAT5 activation. Mol Endocrinol 10:1249–1260

Whitney JA, Gomez M, Sheff D, Kreis TE, Mellman I (1995) Cytoplasmic coat proteins involved in endosome function. Cell 83:703–713

Wiley HS, Burke PM (2001) Regulation of receptor tyrosine kinase signaling by endocytic trafficking. Traffic 2:12–18

Wood TJ, Sliva D, Lobie PE, Goullieux F, Mui AL, Groner B, Norstedt G, Haldosen LA (1997) Specificity of transcription enhancement via the STAT responsive element in the serine protease inhibitor 2.1 promoter. Mol Cell Endocrinol 130:69–81

Yamada K, Lipson KE, Donner DB (1987) Structure and proteolysis of the growth hormone receptor on rat hepatocytes. Biochemistry 26:4438–4443

Yamashiro DJ, Tycko B, Fluss SR, Maxfield FR (1984) Segregation of transferrin to a mildly acidic (pH 6.) para-Golgi compartment in the recycling pathway. Cell 37:789–800

Yaron A, Gonen H, Alkalay I, Hatzubai A, Jung S, Beyth S, Mercurio F, Manning AM, Ciechanover A, Benneriah Y (1997) Inhibition of NF-kappa B cellular function via specific targeting of the I kappa B-ubiquitin ligase. EMBO J 16:6486–6494

Yasukawa H, Misawa H, Sakamoto H, Masuhara M, Sasaki A, Wakioka T, Ohtsuka S, Imaizumi T, Matsuda T, Ihle JN, Yoshimura A (1999) The JAK-binding protein JAB inhibits Janus tyrosine kinase activity through binding in the activation loop. EMBO J 18:1309–1320

Yen CH, Yang YC, Ruscetti SK, Kirken RA, Dai RM, Li CC (2000) Involvement of the ubiquitin-proteasome pathway in the degradation of nontyrosine kinase-type cytokine receptors of IL-9, IL-2, and erythropoietin. J Immunol 165:6372–6380

Yu A, Malek TR (2001) The proteasome regulates receptor-mediated endocytosis of interleukin-2. J Biol Chem 276:381–385

Zhang J-G, Farley A, Nicholson SE, Willson TA, Zugano LM, Simpson RJ, Moritz RL, Cary D, Richardson R, Hausmann G, Kile BJ, Kent SBH, Alexander WS, Metcalf D, Hilton DJ, Nicola NA, Baca M (1999) The conserved SOCS box motif in suppressors of cytokines signalling binds to elongins B and C and may couple bound proteins to proteasomal degradation. Proc Natl Acad Sci USA 96:2071–2076

Zhang Y, Jiang J, Kopchick JJ, Frank SJ (1999) Disulfide linkage of growth hormone (GH) receptors (GHR) reflects GH-induced GHR dimerization—Association of JAK2 with the GHR is enhanced by receptor dimerization. J Biol Chem 274:33072-33084

CTMI (2004) 286:119–148

Clathrin-Independent Endocytosis and Signalling of Interleukin 2 Receptors

IL-2R Endocytosis and Signalling

F. Gesbert* · N. Sauvonnet* · A. Dautry-Varsat (✉)

Unité de Biologie des Interactions Cellulaires – URA CNRS 2582, Institut Pasteur,
25 rue du Docteur Roux, 75724 Paris Cedex 15, France
adautry@pasteur.fr

Abstract Interleukin 2 receptors (IL-2R) belong to the cytokine receptor family and share subunits with other members of the family. They are essential in T cell activation and in maintaining homeostatic immune responses. These receptors do not have an intrinsic kinase activity and use multiple signalling pathways. Their endocytic pathway is different from that of classic growth factor receptors in that it does not follow the classic clathrin-coated pit and vesicle route. After uptake, one of the

---

* contributed equally to this chapter

IL-2R chains, α, recycles to the plasma membrane, whereas the two other chains, β and γ, are targeted to late endosomes/lysosomes and degraded. This involves ubiquitination of the receptor as a sorting signal. Links between the signalling events, internalisation and intracellular sorting of these receptors are reviewed.

1
Introduction

Interleukin (IL) 2 receptors (IL-2R) belong to the cytokine receptor family, which share certain structural and functional features. Originally, the term cytokine was used in the immune system, but many cytokines functions are non-immunologic. Cytokines that bind type I or II receptor families, a classification based on homologies, are secreted factors involved in growth, haematopoiesis, immune regulation, fertility, lactation and embryogenesis. The IL-2R subfamily belongs to the type I group. Most receptors in this group lack intrinsic kinase and other known catalytic domains. They recruit molecules with these properties to transduce signals into the cell.

A unique feature of several members of the family is that they share subunits, which defines subfamilies. The IL-2R, one of the best studied in this group, is composed of three subunits, IL-2Rα (p55, also known as CD25 or Tac), IL-2Rβ (p75, CD122) and IL-2Rγ_c (p64, common γ_c chain, CD132) (reviewed in Gadina et al. 2001; Leonard and Lin 2000). Of the three subunits, only IL-2Rα does not belong to the cytokine family.

The IL-2R subfamily comprises six members: IL-2, IL-4, IL-7, IL-9, IL-15 and IL-21 receptors, which all use the common γ_c chain, in conjunction with ligand-specific chains. Moreover, IL-2 and IL-15 also share the β chain. This particular organisation helps explain some specific or redundant actions of these cytokines.

When the γ_c gene, which is on the X chromosome, is mutated in humans, it results in X-linked severe combined immunodeficiency (XSCID), a profound immunodeficiency characterised by greatly diminished numbers of T and NK cells and the presence of non-functional B cells (reviewed in Fischer 2002; Leonard 2001). Gene therapy trials have been performed to treat XSCID patients (Fischer et al. 2002; Kohn et al. 2003). This illustrates the numerous functions of this family of cytokines on T, NK and B cell development and growth. IL-2R themselves play critical roles on lymphoid lineage cells, particularly activated T lymphocytes and NK cells as they regulate growth, apoptosis and differentiation into effector lymphocytes. They also have played a number of significant roles in the clinic. Their dis-functioning has been proposed to participate in pathogenic states, and conversely, IL-2 has proven useful in the treatment of some cancers and in some cases of HIV infection (reviewed in Gaffen 2001; Waldmann 2002).

IL-2 receptors exist in different forms. The functional forms are either the high-affinity receptor (IL-2Rα, β and γ_c; $K_d \cong$ 10–100 pM), which signals efficiently at biological concentrations of IL-2, or the intermediate-affinity receptor (IL-2Rβ and γ_c; $K_d \cong$ 1 nM), which can also signal. Both the high- and intermediate-affinity receptors are endocytosed. In contrast, IL-2Rα by itself has a low affinity for IL-2 ($K_d \cong$ 10 nM). This low-affinity receptor is expressed under physiological conditions as IL-2Rα is present on activated lymphocytes at much higher levels than IL-2Rβ and γ_c to which it associates to form high-affinity receptors. The sole role of IL-2Rα is in ligand binding; it is an important affinity modulator essential for proper responses and plays a critical role in vivo to sensitise target cells to physiological levels of IL-2. It cannot deliver intracellular signals and is not involved in efficient receptor-mediated endocytosis, whereas IL-2Rβ and γ_c contribute to ligand binding, signal transduction and endocytosis (reviewed in Leonard and Lin 2000; Taniguchi 1995).

IL-2 receptor expression is tightly regulated. The high-affinity receptors are expressed transiently on lymphocytes for a few days after activation, because transcription of the IL-2Rα gene is tightly regulated and is transient. Thus studies of high-affinity functional IL-2R have been performed on activated lymphocytes and a few tumour cell lines that express these receptors.

The three subunits are expressed on the cell surface largely independently of each other in the absence of IL-2, and thus their properties can be studied separately in the absence of IL-2. As is the case for most cytokine receptors, signalling by IL-2 follows ligand-induced oligomerisation of IL-2R subunits. Another important event that follows is endocytosis of IL-2R. Interestingly, both IL-2Rβ and γ_c are efficiently internalised independently of the ligand and of the other chains.

A number of reviews have already discussed signalling by IL-2R. Here, we briefly sum up a large extent of important work on this topic, review what is known on IL-2R endocytosis, which follows a novel pathway and, based on recent work on other receptors following the classic clathrin-dependent pathway, discuss possible links between signalling and endocytosis of IL-2R.

2
Signalling by IL-2 Receptors

The three subunits of the IL-2R participate differently in signalling. The α chain, which is not expressed in resting T lymphocytes and is induced transiently upon activation, functions mainly as an affinity converter. Its cytosolic tail is very short and thus does not, physically, participate in the propagation of the signals. The IL-2Rβ chain, shared with the IL-15 receptor, is a 585-amino acid (aa)-long type I transmembrane protein and has, by far, been the most studied. Its 286-aa-long cytosolic part has been divided into a series of domains, which have been characterised by deletion mutations (Fig. 1). The membrane proximal region contains two short domains (14 aa long) named Box1 and 2. Box 2 encompasses a "serine-rich" domain (S domain) that extends from aa 267 to 322. This domain is followed by an "acidic domain" (A domain, aa 313–382) and the COOH-terminal domain, also called the "proline-rich" domain, which contains the last 147 aa (Fig. 1). The entire cytosolic tail of

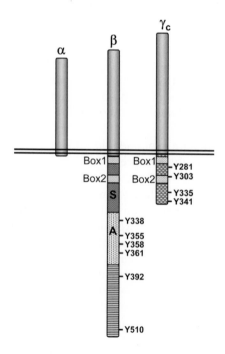

Fig. 1. Scheme of the IL-2R chains cytosolic subdomains and residues involved in signalling

IL-2Rβ contains six tyrosine residues that are putative phosphorylation sites. The IL-2Rγ_c chain, shared by the receptors for interleukin-2, -4, -7, -9, -15 and −21, is a 347-aa-long type I transmembrane receptor. Its 86-aa-long cytosolic tail contains six tyrosine residues, and as for the IL-2Rβ chain, its proximal domain also contains a tandem Box1-Box2 motif. Both IL-2Rβ and γ_c are responsible for signalling, and below we review the cascades activated when IL-2 binds either to the high-affinity receptor, composed of the three chains, or to the intermediate-affinity receptor, composed of IL-2Rβ and γ_c (reviewed in Minami et al. 1993).

2.1
The Jak-STAT Pathway

The Jak-signal transducer and activator of transcription (STAT) pathway is one of the most important signalling cascades activated downstream of cytokine receptors, especially because it creates a rapid link from the plasma membrane to the nucleus (Imada and Leonard 2000). In the case of IL-2 signalling, the activation of the Janus kinases (Jak) 1 and 3 is one of the first events following binding of IL-2 to high- and intermediate-affinity receptors. Deficiency of either Jak3 or Jak1 almost completely abrogates IL-2 signalling and leads to abnormal lymphoid development resulting in SCID syndrome in humans and/or mice (Imada and Leonard 2000; Rodig et al. 1998).

Jak1 and Jak3 bind constitutively to Box 1 and Box 2 of IL-2Rβ and γ_c, respectively (Figs. 1 and 2). Upon ligand-induced heterodimerisation of IL-2Rβ and γ_c, the juxtaposition of Jak1 and Jak3 induces their transphosphorylation and thus their activation. Activated Jaks in turn phosphorylate several tyrosine residues of IL-2Rβ which become targets for signalling molecules with phosphotyrosine-binding motifs (Gaffen 2001). Thus Jak activation constitutes the starting point of parallel cascades in IL-2 signalling. One of these is the STAT pathway involved in lymphocyte proliferation. Upon IL-2 treatment, STAT1, STAT3 and STAT5a and -b can be recruited to phosphotyrosines 338, 392 and 510 of IL-2Rβ, via their src-homology 2 domain (SH2) (Gaffen 2001). This event allows the activated Jaks to phosphorylate the STATs. Phosphorylation of the STATs then induces their dimerisation, activation and translocation to the nucleus, where they can modulate expression of target genes (Fig. 2). Activated STATs, in association with other transcription factors, finally induce the expression of genes involved in cell cycle progression and cell survival (Imada and Leonard 2000; Lin and Leonard 2000). In addition, the STAT pathway regulates the expression of the

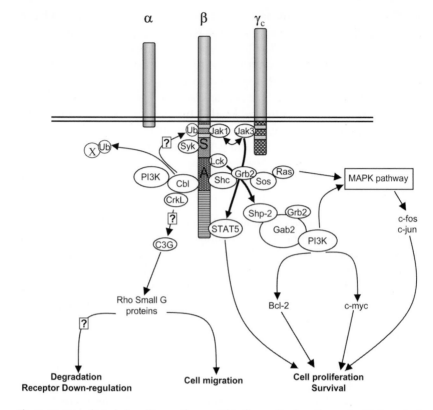

Fig. 2. IL-2-mediated signalling pathways. This figure displays the major IL-2-evoked signalling molecules (see text for details). *?* indicates a link that remains to be clearly established. *X* represents a protein that might be a target for Cbl-mediated ubiquitination

high-affinity IL-2R, by inducing IL-2Rα expression. Furthermore, STAT5 activation plays a role in a feedback loop by inducing the expression of cytokine-inducible SH2-containing protein (CIS) which inhibits the Jak-STAT pathway and might participate in the downmodulation of certain surface receptors (Lin and Leonard 2000).

2.2
Other IL-2-Induced Tyrosine Kinases

Different members of the src-family kinases, in particular $p56^{Lck}$ (Lck) and, in its absence, $p59^{Fyn}$ (Fyn) and $p53^{Lyn}$ (Lyn), bind constitutively to the A region of IL-2Rβ (Fig. 1) (Kobayashi et al. 1993). Upon IL-2 treatment, Lck becomes activated and phosphorylates tyrosines 355, 358, 361, 392 and 510 of IL-2Rβ (Delespine-Carmagnat et al. 1999). The phosphotyrosine residues 392 and 510 are targets for STAT5 recruitment, leading to its phosphorylation independently of Jak3 (Fig. 2; Zhou et al. 2000). However, despite this result, the role of Lck in STAT activation is still a matter of debate. More generally, the function of Lck in IL-2 signalling is not clear, especially because T cells from Lck$^{-/-}$ mice exhibit a normal proliferative response to IL-2 (Molina et al. 1992). It should be noted that this absence of phenotype in cells lacking Lck is probably due to the redundancy of the src-kinases.

Syk is another tyrosine kinase, constitutively associated with the S region of IL-2Rβ, which is activated by IL-2 treatment (Fig. 1). In contrast to Lck, Syk activation is mediated by Jak3 and Jak1 activity (Fig. 2; Zhou et al. 2000). However, Syk is not involved in STAT activation. Although the role of Syk has been associated with c-myc induction and T cell proliferation, the precise function of this kinase is still unclear because Syk$^{-/-}$ mice have a relatively normal IL-2 response (Turner et al. 1995).

2.3
The PI 3-Kinase Pathway

Phosphatidylinositol 3-kinase (PI 3-kinase) is involved in the control of multiple cell processes, such as cell growth, survival and differentiation (Koyasu 2003). The class I PI 3-kinase is composed of two subunits, a regulatory subunit (p85) and a catalytic subunit (p110). This activated enzyme catalyses the phosphorylation of phosphoinositides (PI) generating messengers such as PI 3-phosphate (PI(3)P), PI 3,4-biphosphate (PI(3,4)P$_2$) and PI 3,4,5-triphosphate (PI(3,4,5)P$_3$). The cellular distribution of these lipids may vary. Whereas PI(3,4)P$_2$ and PI(3,4,5)P$_3$ are mainly present at the plasma membrane, PI(3)P is essentially concentrated in endosomal membranes (Czech 2003). PI 3-kinase is also very rapidly induced upon IL-2 treatment, but how it is recruited has been matter of debate because of the lack of PI 3-kinase binding domain in either chain of IL-2R. The current model is that activated Shc-Grb2 complexes recruit the Gab2 adapter to IL-2Rβ, resulting in p85 recruitment and finally PI 3-kinase activation (Gaffen 2001; Gu et al. 2000; see below and Fig. 2). In addition, it has recently been suggested that the upstream molecule involved in PI 3-kinase induction is the tyrosine kinase Syk which would recruit and phosphorylate Shc to IL-2Rβ (Fig. 2; Jiang et al. 2003).

The products of PI 3-kinase, the PIPs, constitute targets for proteins bearing a pleckstrin homology (PH) domain. Protein kinase B (Akt), which is known to induce anti-apoptotic signalling, in particular by inducing bcl-2 expression, belongs to this category (Fig. 2; Gaffen 2001). Through the activation of Akt, PI 3-kinase is also involved in the IL-2-dependent T cell proliferation by activating p70 S6 kinase. Indeed, this kinase was shown to control the translation of certain mRNAs involved in cell division. Another example of the pleiotropic effect of PI 3-kinase is its role on the activation of the mitogen-activated protein kinase kinase (MEK) (Karnitz et al. 1995). The role of MEK, via extracellular signal-regulated kinase Erk, in the phosphorylation and activation of STAT3 makes a link between PI 3-kinase and the STAT pathway (Fung et al. 2003). Thus PI 3-kinase plays a central role in IL-2 signalling.

2.4
The Ras/MAPK Cascade

The Ras proto-oncogene products regulate cell growth in response to a variety of growth factors and are mutated in various cancers. Ras is activated by IL-2 in human T lymphocytes, in a dose-dependent manner (Graves et al. 1992). Deletion studies on the cytosolic tail of IL-2Rβ showed that the A domain is required for Ras activation (Satoh et al. 1992; Figs. 1, 2).

Upon IL-2 stimulation, Shc binds to the phosphorylated tyrosine 338 residue (Evans et al. 1995; Ravichandran and Burakoff 1994) and is then phosphorylated. This Shc phosphorylation creates a docking site for the SH2 domain of the docking protein Grb2, a small protein composed of one SH2 domain surrounded by two SH3 domains. Through its SH3 domains, Grb2 is constitutively associated to various partners, among which is the Ras exchange factor Sos. The recruitment of Sos to the plasma membrane engages the activation of Ras and leads to the activation of the serine/threonine kinase MAPK via the activation of Raf-1 (Karnitz et al. 1995; Fig. 2).

Ultimately, the IL-2-dependent activation of the MAPK cascade leads to the expression of survival- or growth-related genes (such as c-fos, c-jun, bcl2 and bcl-X_L).

2.5
The Gab2/Shp-2 Pathway

It is now well established that many growth factor-induced signalling pathways are regulated by tyrosine phosphorylation. The global level of tyrosine phosphorylation is regulated by protein tyrosine kinases and phosphatases. The functions of protein-tyrosine kinases in IL-2 signalling have been well studied and were described above. More efforts have been aimed at understanding the regulation and the functions of protein tyrosine phosphatases in the past few years. Protein tyrosine phosphatases represent a large superfamily which, as for protein-tyrosine kinases, comprises transmembrane and cytosolic members (Neel et al. 2003).

It was recently shown that Shp-2, a SH2 domain containing cytosolic protein tyrosine phosphatase, is tyrosine phosphorylated and activated in response to IL-2 (Adachi et al. 1997; Gesbert et al. 1998b). The cellular functions regulated by Shp-2 remain largely unknown. It was first described, in PDGF-R-mediated signalling, as an adapter protein responsible for the recruitment of the Grb2/Sos complex and, hence, for the activation of the Ras/MAPK cascade (Bennett et al. 1994). More recent models suggest that Shp-2 phosphatase activity is also required for the regulation of signalling cascades; however, its key substrates are unknown. IL-2-induced activation of Shp-2 was shown to be a Jak-independent mechanism, and a role of Lck/Fyn tyrosine kinases has been suggested (Adachi et al. 1997).

This IL-2-evoked activation of Shp-2 is required to activate the MAPK cascade. The use of a dominant-negative trapping mutant of Shp-2, which has lost the ability to dephosphorylate and remains associated to its substrates, revealed that Shp-2 directly binds to Gab2 and STAT5 and might be responsible for their dephosphorylation (Gu et al. 1998; Yu et al. 2000b). The search for Shp-2 function in cytokine signalling led to the identification of macromolecular complexes. In these, a central position is held by Gab2, a docking protein that has been shown to interact with Grb2, PI 3-kinase and CrkL, in addition to Shp-2 (Crouin et al. 2001; Gesbert et al. 1998b; Gu et al. 1998; Fig. 2). Gab2 is a 97- to 100-kDa protein, which belongs to a family of docking proteins, including Gab1, Gab2, Gab3 and the Drosophila homolog Dos. Gab2 is tyrosine phosphorylated in response to IL-2 and IL-15, but not in response to other cytokine receptors that share IL-2Rγ_c (Brockdorff et al. 2001; Gadina et al. 2000). This would suggest some degree of specificity and probably the requirement of the IL-2Rβ chain in this mechanism. As discussed above, Gab2 may very well be the docking protein required for the recruitment of PI 3-kinase, as the cytosolic part of the IL-2R chains lack a specific binding site for PI 3-kinase (Fig. 2).

Interestingly, although this has not been shown in response to IL-2, it has been reported that Shp-2 regulates RhoA activity (Schoenwaelder 2000). This observation is of particular interest as discussed below. Furthermore, we mentioned above that CrkL is another partner of Gab2 in IL-2 signalling. Although its function remains to be elucidated, it is worth mentioning that this small adaptor protein may provide a link, through its association with the exchange factor C3G, between IL-2R and members of the Rho family of small GTPases, Rac1 and Cdc42.

2.6
Cbl: Docking Protein or Ubiquitin Ligase?

The c-Cbl proto-oncogene was first identified in mice which developed leukaemia in response to an infection by the Cas-Br-M retrovirus. These studies led to the identification of the Cas NS-1 retrovirus which encodes the oncogene v-Cbl (for Casitas B-lineage lymphoma), and provokes pre- and pro-B lymphomas. Further studies showed that v-Cbl is a truncated form of c-Cbl and that overexpression of c-Cbl does not promote tumorigenesis (Langdon et al. 1989). In recent years c-Cbl has been demonstrated to be tyrosine phosphorylated in response to various growth factors and cytokines, including IL-2 (Barber et al. 1997; Bowtell and Langdon 1995; Cory et al. 1995; Gesbert et al. 1998a; Odai et al. 1995).

Despite tremendous efforts, the precise function of Cbl in growth factor signalling remains unclear. The molecular characterisation of Cbl showed that it is composed of several conserved domains. In its N-terminal part it contains a tyrosine kinase-binding domain which was shown to directly bind specific tyrosine-phosphorylated residues on activated tyrosine kinases (Lupher et al. 1998; Miyake et al. 1999). It also contains a Ring finger domain, and this observation led to the discovery that Cbl proteins are ubiquitin ligases (Waterman et al. 1999). In its very C-terminal part, Cbl also contains a ubiquitin-binding domain that might be necessary for its ubiquitin ligase activity. Finally, c-Cbl also contains multiple tyrosine residues, which are phosphorylated and may serve as docking sites for other signalling molecules such as Vav1, PI 3-kinase, CrkL or 14-3-3 (Thien and Langdon 2001; Fig. 2). It is noteworthy that v-Cbl is only composed of the N-terminal tyrosine kinase-binding domain and thus does not exhibit ubiquitin ligase activity, nor can it bind to the majority of the partners found associated with c-Cbl.

The function of c-Cbl in IL-2 signalling has not been determined so far. It might play a role in the downregulation of the receptor through ubiquitination and subsequent degradation as it does in the case of the EGF-R, although the exact mechanism is still a matter of debate (Duan et al. 2003; Waterman et al. 1999). However, c-Cbl might also play an important role as an adaptor protein, as it was demonstrated to bind Grb2, Shc, PI 3-kinase, and CrkL in IL-2-stimulated T lymphocytes.

3
Endocytosis of IL-2 Receptors

IL-2R are among the few physiological markers which allowed the definition of a clathrin-independent receptor-mediated endocytosis pathway. Indeed, the most extensively characterised mechanism of endocytosis is clathrin mediated. Irrefutable evidence has accumulated over the years that clathrin-coated pits form at the plasma membrane, bud and form clathrin-coated vesicles, which transport membrane receptors and their ligands as well as solutes into the cells. For many years, the intense interest in this pathway overshadowed the possibility that other endocytic pathways might exist. Recently, however, the existence of alternative pathways has become widely accepted, although the molecular mechanisms involved are still far from being understood. In fact, it turns out that there may be several clathrin-independent endocytosis pathways.

3.1
Clathrin-Independent Endocytosis

Along the years, while the now classic clathrin-dependent endocytosis pathway was studied, other endocytic pathways which do not use clathrin were also observed (Dautry-Varsat 2001). However, two difficulties slowed down progress for a long time. One was the dearth of specific markers which are strictly internalised independently of coated pits and vesicles. The other difficulty was finding ways to perturb the classic pathway specifically. Interestingly, it is the major progress made in the last few years in identifying the molecular machinery of the classic pathway that allowed the design of several specific tools to specifically inhibit it. Thus several specific markers of clathrin-independent endocytosis have been found recently and have established the physiological relevance of these alternate routes.

Clathrin-independent endocytosis includes the constitutive pinocytosis pathway as well as endocytosis mediated by caveolae and lipid microdomains. We will briefly review clathrin-independent receptor-mediated endocytosis and will not discuss phagocytosis and macropinocytosis which are not relevant here.

Caveolae were observed long ago and their potential role in endocytosis was debated. Caveolae represent a subset of lipid microdomains which are further characterised by the presence of the protein caveolin (van Deurs et al. 2003). Lipid microdomains are diverse dynamic membrane domains, enriched in cholesterol and glycosphingolipids, which are intensively studied and debated (reviewed in Brown and London 2000; Simons and Ehehalt 2002). Biochemically, they can be enriched from cell extracts as low-density detergent-resistant membranes (DRM, also called rafts). Several recent reports show that caveolae mediate endocytosis by a process involving dynamin, as is the case for the classic pathway (for recent reviews, see Kurzchalia and Parton 1999; Nabi and Le 2003; Schlegel and Lisanti 2001; van Deurs et al. 2003). In contrast to clathrin-mediated endocytosis, caveolae-mediated endocytosis appears to be a triggered event. Indeed, for instance, entry of the virus SV40 which is taken up via caveolae has been characterised. Triggering of its uptake can occur by clustering of lipid microdomains components as glycosyphophatidylinositol (GPI)-anchored proteins and MHC class 1 molecules, to which SV40 binds, on the plasma membrane. The clusters are sequestered into caveolae, and a signal transduction cascade is initiated (reviewed in Pelkmans and Helenius 2003).

An interesting hypothesis is that an important function of caveolin would be to stabilise a subset of lipid rafts and to protect them against internalisation. Following this hypothesis, one can propose that caveolae and lipid microdomains mediate a common endocytic pathway, defined by its clathrin independence, its dynamin dependence and its sensitivity to cholesterol depletion (Nabi and Le 2003; van Deurs et al. 2003). Several arguments are in favour of this hypothesis: Autocrine motility factor, for instance, is internalised in caveolae but is still internalised in cells expressing few cell surface caveolae; cholera toxin is internalised partly via caveolae and is still internalised in cells not expressing caveolae and SV40 is internalised more efficiently in cells from caveolin-1 knock-out mice (Nabi and Le 2003; van Deurs et al. 2003). It is noteworthy that in addition to these, other clathrin-independent pathways may also exist.

3.2
The Initial Steps of IL-2R Endocytosis

Initial studies indicating that IL-2R were internalised independently of clathrin-coated structures used pharmacological methods to inhibit the classic pathway (potassium depletion, cytosol acidification and treatment with chlorpromazine) in lymphocytes. Treatments which inhibited internalisation of transferrin, which follows the classic pathway, by 90%, inhibited internalisation of IL-2 bound to high-affinity receptors (IL-2Rα, β and γ_c) by less than 30%. The same result was obtained, studying IL-2Rβ internalisation using bound monoclonal antibodies (Subtil et al. 1994). Thus, when clathrin-coated vesicle formation was impaired, IL-2 was still internalised. The small inhibition observed could be due to the fact that these treatments, which are not specific, could also affect the IL-2 pathway. Alternatively, it could suggest that IL-2 and its high-affinity receptors were internalised by a new pathway and partly by the classic pathway. With the recent availability of molecular inhibitors of the clathrin-dependent pathway (Dautry-Varsat 2001), the pathway followed by IL-2Rβ was investigated in transfected non-lymphocytic cells. IL-2Rβ was efficiently internalised despite the selective inhibition of clathrin-dependent endocytosis by dominant-negative mutants of Eps15. This protein is essential for the formation of clathrin-coated pits and vesicles, and deletion mutants have been shown to specifically prevent the formation of coated pits (Benmerah et al. 1999). In contrast, overexpression of dominant-negative mutants of dynamin 1 or 2 inhibited IL-2Rβ uptake (Lamaze et al. 2001 and unpublished results). In lymphocytes which are naturally devoid of caveolae, IL-2Rβ was observed to be localised in areas of the plasma membrane which do not contain clathrin-coated structures (Fig. 3) and was enriched in lipid microdomains, as assessed biochemically. IL-2Rα, which by itself is not efficiently internalised, was also reported to be clustered on the surface of lymphocytes in a cholesterol-dependent way, independently of IL-2Rβ (Vereb et al. 2000). Also, nystatin, which depletes cholesterol, inhibits IL-2Rβ internalisation in lymphocytes but not that of the classic pathway marker transferrin (unpublished results). Clathrin-independent internalisation of IL-2R is thus independent of caveolae, appears to involve membrane microdomains and, importantly, is a rapid and efficient process. In agreement with these endocytic properties, IL-2Rβ and γ_c do not contain a classic coated-pit localisation signal. Each chain contains weak motifs which promote entry in an additive way; one is in the trans-

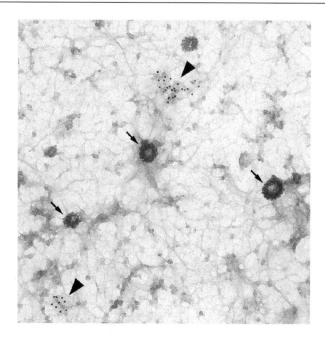

Fig. 3. Clathrin-independent internalisation of IL-2 receptor. The IL-2Rβ chains were stained at the cell surface of T lymphocytes with gold-labelled antibodies and observed by electron microscopy. IL-2Rβ (*arrowheads*) were not found in clathrin-coated pits (*arrows*) or clathrin flat lattices as shown by quantitative analysis. (Reprinted from Lamaze et al. 2001, with permission from Elsevier)

membrane domain of IL-2Rβ and the others are located in the cytosolic tails (Morelon and Dautry-Varsat 1998; Subtil and Dautry-Varsat 1998).

Another interesting aspect concerns the potential role of the cytoskeleton in the IL-2R pathway. The role of the microtubule cytoskeleton in the coated pit pathway has been recently investigated, following several earlier observations (Rappoport et al. 2003 and references therein). With total internal reflection microscopy, clathrin spots have been observed to move along the microtubule cytoskeleton parallel to the cell surface. In agreement with this, disrupting the microtubule cytoskeleton with nocodazole in lymphocytes inhibited transferrin internalisation via coated structures. Interestingly, in these cells, which express IL-2R, internalisation of IL-2 bound to the high-affinity receptors or of IL-2Rβ by itself was not affected. However, when a coated pit localisation signal was added to IL-2Rβ, disruption of the microtubules inhibited internalisation of this chimera (Subtil and Dautry-Varsat 1997).

The role of the actin cytoskeleton and of small GTPases of the Rho family has been studied in some detail. These have been involved in several endocytic pathways (Ellis and Mellor 2000; Hall 1998). Regarding the classic pathway, it has been shown that RhoA and Rac1 control the formation of clathrin-coated vesicles at the plasma membrane of HeLa cells (Lamaze et al. 1996). Interestingly, the pathway followed by IL-2Rβ is regulated differently. Overexpression of activated RhoA did not inhibit IL-2Rβ internalisation, whereas it prevented transferrin uptake. Overexpression of the inactive GDP-RhoA mutant or of Rho GDI inhibited IL-2Rβ but not transferrin internalisation (Lamaze et al. 2001; Sabharanjak et al. 2002). It is noteworthy that the clathrin-independent pathway followed by GPI-anchored proteins, which are concentrated in caveolae, does not appear to be regulated by RhoA (Sabharanjak et al. 2002).

As discussed above, functional IL-2R as well as the kinases and adaptor molecules necessary for IL-2 signalling are expressed in activated lymphocytes and a few lymphocytic cell lines. The number of receptors expressed is very low (usually 3,000–5,000 per cell), and these cells are difficult to study (they are small and very difficult to transfect). As a result, a number of studies have been performed in non-lymphocytic cells transfected with one chain. In this context, it is important to check the properties of these chains independently of the others and of the signalling molecules.

Whether IL-2 is bound to the high-affinity receptor, composed of the three chains, or to the intermediate-affinity receptor, composed of IL-2Rβ and γ_c, its internalisation is similar. IL-2Rβ or γ_c, when transfected alone in cells not expressing the other chain, are internalised at a rate of about half of that of IL-2 bound to the receptors. An interesting model was provided by an Epstein-Barr virus-transformed B lymphocytic cell line established from a patient with X-linked immunodeficiency. The mutation in IL-2Rγ_c in this case resulted in a deletion of the cytosolic tail of IL-2Rγ_c, but the transmembrane and extracellular domain were expressed on the cell surface and associated with IL-2Rα and β to bind IL-2 with the normal high affinity. In this case, IL-2 was internalised at about half the rate of normal high-affinity receptors, for example, that of IL-2Rβ alone. Therefore, the association of IL-2Rβ and γ_c results in an increased internalisation efficiency (Morelon et al. 1996). Because IL-2Rγ_c is largely responsible for the initiation of IL-2 signalling, this result can be interpreted in two ways. One interesting possibility is that molecules involved in IL-2 signalling could affect receptor internalisation. Another possibility is that because both IL-2Rβ and γ_c are endowed with internalisation properties, their signals could add up to render the process more efficient.

An important question concerns the internalisation pathway of high-affinity receptors. The clathrin-independent pathway has been studied in detail with molecular tools in non-lymphocytic cell lines transfected to express IL-2Rβ. Therefore, one may wonder whether high-affinity receptors follow only this pathway, as is the case for IL-2Rβ, or whether they could also be internalised via coated pits, specially in the light of the recent data concerning TGF-β receptors (Di Guglielmo et al. 2003). In view of the studies on high-affinity IL-2R using drugs that prevent the clathrin-dependent pathway or studying the role of the microtubule cytoskeleton (see above), it appears that functional high-affinity IL-2R also follow the clathrin-independent pathway. However, because these treatments partially inhibited IL-2 uptake (Subtil and Dautry-Varsat 1997), the possibility that high-affinity IL-2R are internalised partly by the classic pathway cannot be completely ruled out.

3.3
Endocytosis and IL-2 Signalling

3.3.1
Putative IL-2 Signalling Factors Involved in IL-2R Endocytosis

Different results are in agreement with an involvement of IL-2 signalling factors in IL-2R endocytosis: (i) the internalisation kinetics of the high affinity IL-2R are twice as fast as those of IL-2Rβ or IL-2Rγ$_c$ alone (Morelon et al. 1996); (ii) the truncation of the cytoplasmic tail of IL-2Rγ$_c$, which is absolutely required for IL-2 signalling, results in slower internalisation kinetics of JL-2R as does the absence of IL-2 (Morelon et al. 1996; Yu et al. 2000a); (iii) the rate of IL-2R internalisation is twice as fast in lymphoid cells as in other cell types incapable of promoting IL-2 signalling (Yu et al. 2000a).

In particular, this last result prompted Yu et al. to test the role of tyrosine kinases, largely involved in IL-2 signalling (Yu et al. 2000a). The tyrosine kinase inhibitor genistein was able to partially inhibit IL-2R endocytosis (by a factor of 2), but only in lymphoid cells. Because the Jaks are essentially expressed in lymphoid cells and are involved early in IL-2 signalling, they could represent good tyrosine kinase candidates. However, it should be noted that transfection of either Jak1 or Jak3 in epithelial cells was not sufficient to increase IL-2R internalisation in these cells

(Yu et al. 2000a). Nevertheless, this result does not eliminate the Jaks as kinase candidates involved in IL-2R internalisation.

3.3.1.1
PI 3-Kinase

PI 3-kinase is involved in phagocytosis and also in receptor-mediated endocytosis (Takenawa and Itoh 2001). PI 3-kinase does not seem to be involved in all clathrin-dependent internalisation, because it has no effect on transferrin receptor endocytosis, but it is involved in some cases. In particular, it was shown that β-adrenergic receptor endocytosis depends on PI 3-kinase by recruiting AP-2 to the receptor-β-arrestin complex (Naga Prasad et al. 2002). Another example is the AP-2-independent endocytosis of class I major histocompatibility (MHC-I) triggered by HIV-1 Nef (Blagoveshchenskaya et al. 2002). It was shown that Nef activates PI 3-kinase, catalysing the production of $PI(3,4,5)P_3$, which in turn recruits ARNO and finally induces Arf6 activation that is required for MHC-I endocytosis. Because PI 3-kinase is a key actor in IL-2 signalling (see above) and plays a role in distinct endocytosis mechanisms, this lipid kinase could be involved in IL-2R endocytosis. Our preliminary results showing that the PI 3-kinase inhibitor LY294002 affects IL-2R endocytosis are in good agreement with this hypothesis (our unpublished data).

3.3.1.2
Lck, Src Kinases and Lipid Microdomains

Our results suggest that IL-2Rβ endocytosis involves lipid microdomains (see above and Lamaze et al. 2001). Microdomains are known to act as signalling platforms which facilitate intramolecular association and the propagation of signal transduction cascades especially in lymphocytes (Brown and London 2000). The recruitment of IL-2Rβ in lipid microdomains reinforces the potential links between endocytosis and IL-2 signalling. Different groups have investigated the role of lipid microdomains in IL-2 signalling (Goebel et al. 2002; Marmor and Julius 2001; Matko et al. 2002), however their results are sometimes conflicting. Nevertheless, two reports have shown that disruption of lipid microdomains by β-methylcyclodextrin treatment, depleting the cells of cholesterol, attenuated the IL-2-induced tyrosine phosphorylation (Goebel et al. 2002; Matko et al. 2002). Src kinases, such as Lck, are associated constitutively to IL-2Rβ (see above), and some are concentrated in lipid microdomains via their fatty acid modification. Thus Lck represents a good tyrosine kinase candidate involved in both IL-2R endocytosis and IL-2 signalling. However, its role in internalisation is difficult to predict because Lck has been negatively involved in receptor-mediated endocytosis of CD4 (cluster of differentiation antigen 4) (Pelchen-Matthews et al. 1998). Indeed, CD4 internalisation was shown to be activated in the absence of Lck. The association of CD4 with Lck in lipid microdomains hides a classic di-leucine endocytosis signal present in CD4, thereby blocking its clathrin-dependent internalisation (Pitcher et al. 1999).

3.3.2
IL-2 Signalling Factors Activated by IL-2R Endocytosis

Another question concerns the possibility that molecules involved in the IL-2 cascade could signal after receptor endocytosis. This phenomenon has been clearly demonstrated in the case of the EGF-R (Sorkin and Von Zastrow 2002) after years of controversy, but so far, nothing is known for IL-2R. This is difficult to investigate because the endocytic signals present in IL-2Rβ or γ_c match within regions essential for IL-2 signalling, thereby preventing the construction of mutants supposed to affect only endocytosis. However, data obtained for other receptors showed that several IL-2 signalling molecules such as Grb2, Shc, Gab2, Ras, PI 3-kinase and MEK can be present in endosomes (Sorkin and Von Zastrow 2002). This may suggest that at least partial activation of Ras-MAPK, Gab2-Shp-2 and PI 3-kinase pathways could take place once high-affinity IL-2R are endocytosed. Such may also be the case for the complete activation of the STATs. Indeed, it was shown that the clathrin-dependent endocytosis of EGF-R and the lipid microdomain-dependent endocytosis of IFNγ-1R were required for the translocation to the nucleus of STAT3 and STAT1, respectively (Bild et al. 2002; Subramaniam and Johnson 2002). Last but not least, the observation that the two endocytic pathways taken by TGF-β lead to different fates (Di Guglielmo et al. 2003), either a rapid downmodulation of the receptor or intracellular signalling, might also apply to the IL-2R. The possibility remains that, in the presence of IL-2, part of the high-affinity receptor might be internalised by a clathrin-dependent pathway, enabling some intracellular signalling and part by a lipid microdomain way, allowing rapid degradation of IL-2Rβ and γ_c.

3.4
Intracellular Sorting of IL-2R

3.4.1
IL-2Rβ Sorting Signal to Late Endosomes/Lysosomes

As many endocytosed growth factors, IL-2 is degraded in late endo-
somes/lysosomes. The fate of the three receptor's chains, however, is different. Once they are internalised, associated in high-affinity receptors,
IL-2Rβ and γ_c are also sorted to late endosomes/lysosomes and degraded, while IL-2Rα is recycled to the plasma membrane (Hémar et al.
1995). Each of the two chains, IL-2Rβ or γ_c, when transfected by itself, is
also sorted to these degradation compartments (Fig. 4). In lymphocytes
IL-2Rβ and γ_c were observed to be colocalised with transferrin, a marker
of early and recycling endosomes, by confocal microscopy, a few minutes after uptake. Later on, they colocalised with Rab7, a late endosome
marker. Thus these receptors appear to follow the usual endocytic route,
despite their non-classic internalisation pathway. However, considering
the experimental difficulties (lymphocytes are small cells and express
few receptors), it is impossible to rule out that part of the receptors are
sorted to other compartments. Indeed, other markers following a clathrin-independent pathway (SV40, GPI-anchored protein, autocrine motility factor) have been reported to be transported to the Golgi, the ER or
the newly described caveosomes, with discussions still remaining in
some cases (Johannes and Lamaze 2002; Nabi and Le 2003; Nichols

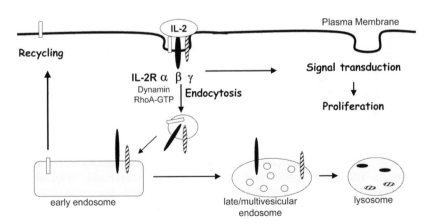

Fig. 4. Major intracellular events induced in lymphocytes upon IL-2 treatment

2002; Pelkmans and Helenius 2003; Sabharanjak et al. 2002; van Deurs et al. 2003). Interestingly, SV40 in cells devoid of caveolin goes partly to caveosomes and partly to endosomes.

The sorting of IL-2Rβ was studied in more detail. It contains in its intracellular tail a 10-amino acid signal, which is necessary for its sorting from early to late endosomes (Subtil et al. 1997; Subtil et al. 1998). Deletion of this signal prevents IL-2Rβ targeting to degradation compartments. This signal, when grafted on a chimeric receptor constructed to be internalised via the classic coated pit pathway, is sufficient to target it away from recycling to late endosomes and lysosomes. It is noteworthy that this sequence is a sorting motif and is not, by itself, an internalisation signal.

3.4.2
Ubiquitination-Dependent Sorting

Further characterisation of the sorting processes followed by IL-2 receptors led to the demonstration that it is dependent on the ubiquitination machinery. The use of a thermo-sensitive cell line, which is defective at a non-permissive temperature, for the ubiquitin-activating enzymes suggested that ubiquitination is required for the sorting of the internalised receptors towards late endosomes/lysosomes. When it could not be ubiquitinated, IL-2Rβ accumulated in early endosomes (Rocca et al. 2001).

Recently, ubiquitination has turned out to have several important, previously unknown, functions in various aspects of cell biology. Ubiquitin is a 76-amino acid protein that is highly conserved in eucaryotes. Ubiquitination consists in the covalent conjugation of ubiquitin on lysine residues of other proteins. This process takes place at the end of a cascade which requires the participation of three types of enzymes. First, E1 ubiquitin-activating enzyme, second, ubiquitin-conjugating enzyme (E2) and third, an E3 ubiquitin ligase (Weissman 2001). Endogenous proteins can be conjugated to a single ubiquitin, termed mono-ubiquitination, or to more than one ubiquitin, each on a different lysine residue, termed multi-ubiquitination. These ubiquitins may themselves serve as conjugation sites, thus creating poly-ubiquitinated chains. Poly-ubiquitination of Lys-48 mediates the best-characterised function of ubiquitin, which targets proteins to the proteasome. Mono-ubiquitination of proteins has been reported to regulate distinct cellular functions. In mammalian cells, it has been shown that plasma membrane-anchored proteins are ubiquitinated, and these events regulate their endocytic transport and their sorting towards lysosomal degradation. It was initially reported in yeast that mono-ubiquitination is sufficient to target proteins to early endosomes (Hicke and Riezman 1996). The internalisation process seems to be regulated by the sole ubiquitin moiety. This mechanism has been shown with chimeric constructs (Haglund et al. 2003). It is noteworthy that a di-leucine motif has been identified in the ubiquitin sequence (Nakatsu et al. 2000). This signal is supposed to be able, by itself, to mediate endocytosis of plasma membrane proteins when fused to the cytosolic tail.

On the other hand, a growing number of reports have proposed that mono-ubiquitination serves as a recognition signal by proteins which belong to the endocytic and sorting machinery (Polo et al. 2002; Shih et al. 2002). Several protein motifs have been shown to specifically bind ubiquitin. First ubiquitin associated (UBA) were described as they were found in proteins involved in ubiquitination/de-ubiquitination processes (Hofmann and Bucher 1996). Second, ubiquitin interacting motif (UIM), that binds directly to mono-ubiquitinated proteins and is ubiquitinated itself (Polo et al. 2002; Shih et al. 2002). Third, the CUE domain, which has been identified by database searches and was first identified in the yeast Cue1 protein (Shih et al. 2003).

One mechanism was proposed recently in the case of the clathrin-dependent internalisation of the EGF-R. The Eps15 protein contains a UIM domain (Klapisz et al. 2002; Polo et al. 2002). Through the ubiquitin-UIM interaction, Eps15 recruits the tagged receptor to coated pits, by interacting with the AP2-clathrin complex, and would thus direct the receptor towards internalisation.

Hrs is another protein that contains a UIM motif and is involved in early endosome sorting (Raiborg et al. 2002; Shih et al. 2002). It is the mammalian homologue of the yeast vps27 protein which was shown to be required in the vacuolar membrane transport machinery. Hrs recruits clathrin to endosomes and may represent one of the major partners involved in endocytic sorting. Furthermore, Hrs contains a FYVE domain which has the ability to specifically interact with PI(3)P that is enriched in early endosomes (Stenmark and Aasland 1999). Recently, a major role was proposed for Hrs in the regulation of the multi-vesicular endosome formation through recruitment of the endosomal sorting complexes required for transport (ESCRT) machinery to endosomes. Three complexes, ESCRT-I, -II and –III, discovered in yeast, function sequentially in recruiting ubiquitinated cargoes and sorting to the MVE machinery (Babst et al. 2002a; Babst et al. 2002b; Katzmann et al. 2001). A role for

Hrs as an adaptor linking ubiquitinated cargoes to ESCRT-I is presently a matter of debate.

Hrs has been shown to be tyrosyl phosphorylated in response to various stimuli, including EGF, PDGF and IL-2 (Asao et al. 1997; Komada and Kitamura 1995). Hrs belongs to a family of proteins which contain a so-called VHS domain (Vps27/Hrs/STAM). This domain, in tandem with the UIM motif, would allow specific binding to ubiquitin (Mizuno et al. 2003). Interestingly, the STAM2 protein has been shown to participate in IL-2 signalling, and its overexpression leads to an increased IL-2 mediated expression of c-myc (Tanaka et al. 1999). STAM2 was first identified as a major tyrosine-phosphorylated protein associated with Hrs, and it has been reported to be phosphorylated in response to IL-2.

Studies performed on EGF-R sorting showed that overexpression of Hrs or STAM leads to similar phenotypes: accumulation of ubiquitinated proteins, accumulation of ligand-activated receptors and enlargement of the cells. Deletion mutants of STAM2 unable to bind Hrs showed a clear decrease of receptor degradation but not receptor internalisation rate, supporting the function of these molecules in the sorting towards degradation of growth factor receptors (Komada and Kitamura 1995; Mizuno et al. 2003; Raiborg et al. 2002).

Most of the studies performed on these molecules were done on receptors which follow the conventional clathrin-dependent pathways. It is not yet known whether these molecules play a role in clathrin-independent endocytosis and sorting.

As is the case for phosphorylation events which are regulated by kinases and phosphatases, ubiquitin can be removed by de-ubiquitinating enzymes. The role of these enzymes still remains controversial. However, it has been suggested, from studies in yeast, that de-ubiquitination may occur either to regulate ligand-induced receptor degradation or to regulate sorting to multi-vesicular endosomes as de-ubiquitination might be required to enter these endosomes (Amerik et al. 2000; Dupre and Haguenauer-Tsapis 2001).

It is noteworthy that an IL-2 induced de-ubiquitinating enzyme, DUB-2, has been described. The overexpression of DUB-2 has been shown to prolong IL-2 signalling and would thus suggest a role in the regulation of receptor downregulation, although this remains to be established (Migone et al. 2001; Zhu 1997).

As far as IL-2 receptor endocytosis and sorting is concerned, it was shown that the IL-2Rβ chain is mono-ubiquitinated in vivo. Lysine residues are the usual targets of ubiquitination. Mutation of the lysine residues, located in the degradation signal of the IL-2Rβ chain transferred to a chimera, impaired its correct sorting and caused its accumulation in early recycling endosomes, whereas it did not modify its internalisation rate (Rocca et al. 2001). The role of ubiquitination under IL-2 signalling is currently being investigated. So far, the molecules that regulate ubiquitination of IL-2Rβ and the ubiquitination-dependent sorting of the receptor have not been characterised. In agreement with the signalling pathways mentioned above, the Cbl/Dub2 pair appears to be the best candidate to regulate the ubiquitination/de-ubiquitination of the IL-2R.

4
Conclusion

For many years, it was considered that endocytosis of growth factor receptors only serves to downregulate and control their expression at the cell surface and that signalling occurred only at the plasma membrane. In recent years, it has clearly been shown that this is not true: Endocytosis and signalling of growth factor receptors which follow the classic clathrin-coated pit pathway are clearly intricate. Concerning IL-2 receptors, taken together, several reports in the literature suggest that signalling might affect their endocytosis and intracellular sorting. More generally, little is known for receptors following clathrin-independent pathways. The molecular mechanisms underlying the initial steps of their internalisation and the regulatory molecules involved are mostly unknown. Their intracellular destinations (Golgi, ER, endosomes, caveosomes...) are intensively studied and may differ. Signalling could occur both at the cell surface and in some of these intracellular compartments. On the other hand, signalling after ligand binding could also affect the trafficking and intracellular destinations of these receptors.

Hopefully, an equivalent review in a few years can provide most of the answers to these questions concerning the clathrin-independent pathways. This is a challenge for future research.

Acknowledgements Work in the authors' laboratory is supported by Association pour la Recherche sur le Cancer. We apologise to our colleagues whose work was omitted, or quoted only in reviews, owing to space constraints.

References

Adachi M, Ishino M, Torigoe T, Minami Y, Matozaki T, Miyazaki T, Taniguchi T, Hinoda Y, and Imai K (1997) Interleukin-2 induces tyrosine phosphorylation of SHP-2 through IL-2 receptor beta chain. Oncogene 14:1629–1633

Amerik AY, Nowak J, Swaminathan S, and Hochstrasser M (2000) The Doa4 deubiquitinating enzyme is functionally linked to the vacuolar protein-sorting and endocytic pathways. Mol Biol Cell 11:3365–3380

Asao H, Sasaki Y, Arita T, Tanaka N, Endo K, Kasai H, Takeshita T, Endo Y, Fujita T, and Sugamura K (1997) Hrs is associated with STAM, a signal-transducing adaptor molecule. Its suppressive effect on cytokine-induced cell growth. J Biol Chem 272:32785–32791

Babst M, Katzmann DJ, Estepa-Sabal EJ, Meerloo T, and Emr SD (2002a) Escrt-III: an endosome-associated heterooligomeric protein complex required for MVB sorting. Dev Cell 3:271–282

Babst M, Katzmann DJ, Snyder WB, Wendland B, and Emr SD (2002b) Endosome-associated complex, ESCRT-II, recruits transport machinery for protein sorting at the multivesicular body. Dev Cell 3:283–289

Barber DL, Mason JM, Fukazawa T, Reedquist KA, Druker BJ, Band H, and D'Andrea AD (1997) Erythropoietin and interleukin-3 activate tyrosine phosphorylation of CBL and association with CRK adaptor proteins. Blood 89:3166–3174

Benmerah A, Lamaze C, Bayrou M, Cerf-Bensussan N, and Dautry-Varsat A (1999) Inhibition of clathrin-coated pit assemby by an Eps15 mutant. J Cell Sci 112:1303–1311

Bennett AM, Tang TL, Sugimoto S, Walsh CT, and Neel BG (1994) Protein-tyrosine-phosphatase SHPTP2 couples platelet-derived growth factor receptor beta to Ras. Proc Natl Acad Sci U S A 91:7335–7339

Bild AH, Turkson J, and Jove R (2002) Cytoplasmic transport of Stat3 by receptor-mediated endocytosis. EMBO J 21:3255–3263

Blagoveshchenskaya AD, Thomas L, Feliciangeli SF, Hung CH, and Thomas G (2002) HIV-1 nef downregulates MHC-I by a PACS-1- and PI3K-regulated ARF6 endocytic pathway. Cell 111:853–866

Bowtell DD, and Langdon WY (1995) The protein product of the c-cbl oncogene rapidly complexes with the EGF receptor and is tyrosine phosphorylated following EGF stimulation. Oncogene 11:1561–1567

Brockdorff JL, Gu H, Mustelin T, Kaltoft K, Geisler C, Ropke C, and Odum N (2001) Gab2 is phosphorylated on tyrosine upon interleukin-2/interleukin-15 stimulation in mycosis-fungoides-derived tumor T cells and associates inducibly with SHP-2 and Stat5a. Exp Clin Immunogenet 18:86–95

Brown DA, and London E (2000) Structure and function of sphingolipid- and cholesterol-rich membrane rafts. J Biol Chem 275:17221–17224

Cory GO, Lovering RC, Hinshelwood S, MacCarthy-Morrogh L, Levinsky RJ, and Kinnon C (1995) The protein product of the c-cbl protooncogene is phosphorylated after B cell receptor stimulation and binds the SH3 domain of Bruton's tyrosine kinase. J Exp Med 182:611–615

Crouin C, Arnaud M, Gesbert F, Camonis J, and Bertoglio J (2001) A yeast two-hybrid study of human p97/Gab2 interactions with its SH2 domain-containing binding partners. FEBS Lett 495:148–153

Czech MP (2003) Dynamics of phosphoinositides in membrane retrieval and insertion. Annu Rev Physiol 65:791–815.

Dautry-Varsat A (2001) Clathrin-independent endocytosis. In: Marsh M (ed) Clathrin-independent endocytosis. Oxford University Press, Oxford, pp 26–57

Delespine-Carmagnat M, Bouvier G, Allée G, Fagard R, and Bertoglio J (1999) Biochemical analysis of interleukin-2 receptor β chain phosphorylation by p56[llck]. FEBS Lett 447:241–246

Di Guglielmo GM, Le Roy C, Goodfellow AF, and Wrana JL (2003) Distinct endocytic pathways regulate TGF-b receptor signalling and turnover. Nat Cell Biol 5:410–421

Duan L, Miura Y, Dimri M, Majumder B, Dodge IL, Reddi AL, Ghosh A, Fernandes N, Zhou P, Mullane-Robinson K, Rao N, Donoghue S, Rogers RA, Bowtell D, Naramura M, Gu H, Band V, and Band H (2003) Cbl-mediated ubiquitinylation is required for lysosomal sorting of epidermal growth factor receptor but is dispensable for endocytosis. J Biol Chem 278:28950–28960.

Dupre S, and Haguenauer-Tsapis R (2001) Deubiquitination step in the endocytic pathway of yeast plasma membrane proteins: crucial role of Doa4p ubiquitin isopeptidase. Mol Cell Biol 21:4482–4494

Ellis S, and Mellor H (2000) Regulation of endocytic traffic by Rho family GTPases. Trends Cell Biol 10:85–88

Evans GA, Goldsmith MA, Johnston JA, Xu W, Weiler SR, Erwin R, Howard OM, Abraham RT, O'Shea JJ, Greene WC, and et al. (1995) Analysis of interleukin-2-dependent signal transduction through the Shc/Grb2 adapter pathway. Interleukin-2-dependent mitogenesis does not require Shc phosphorylation or receptor association. J Biol Chem 270:28858–28863

Fischer A (2002) Primary immunodeficiency diseases : natural mutant models for the study of the immune system. Scand J Immunol 55:238–241

Fischer A, Hacein-Bey S, and Cavazzana-Calvo M (2002) Gene therapy of severe combined immunodeficiencies. Nat Rev Immunol 2:615–621.

Fung MM, Rohwer F, and McGuire KL (2003) IL-2 activation of a PI3K-dependent STAT3 serine phosphorylation pathway in primary human T cells. Cell Signal 15:625–636

Gadina M, Sudarshan C, Visconti R, Zhou YJ, Gu H, Neel BG, and O'Shea JJ (2000) The docking molecule Gab2 is induced by lymphocyte activation and is involved in signaling by interleukin-2 and interleukin-15 but not other common gamma chain-using cytokines. J Biol Chem 275:26959–26966

Gadina M, Hilton D, Johnston JA, Morinobu A, Lighvani A, Zhou Y-J, Visconti R, and O'Shea JJ (2001) Signaling by type I and II cytokine receptors : Ten years after. Curr Opin Immunol 13:363–373

Gaffen SL (2001) Signaling domains of the interleukin 2 receptor. Cytokine 14:63–77

Gesbert F, Garbay C, and Bertoglio J (1998a) Interleukin-2 stimulation induces tyrosine phosphorylation of p120-Cbl and CrkL and formation of multimolecular signaling complexes in T lymphocytes and natural killer cells. J Biol Chem 237:3986–3993

Gesbert F, Guenzi C, and Bertoglio J (1998b) A new tyrosine-phosphorylated 97-kDa adaptor protein mediates interleukin-2-induced association of SHP-2 with p85-phosphatidylinositol 3-kinase in human T lymphocytes. J Biol Chem 273:18273–18281

Goebel J, Forrest K, Morford L, and Roszman TL (2002) Differential localization of IL-2- and -15 receptor chains in membrane rafts of human T cells. J Leukoc Biol 72:199–206

Graves JD, Downward J, Izquierdo-Pastor M, Rayter S, Warne PH, and Cantrell DA (1992) The growth factor IL-2 activates p21ras proteins in normal human T lymphocytes. J Immunol 148:2417–2422

Gu H, Pratt JC, Burakoff SJ, and Neel BG (1998) Cloning of p97/Gab2, the major SHP2-binding protein in hematopoietic cells, reveals a novel pathway for cytokine-induced gene activation. Mol Cell 2:729–740

Gu H, Maeda H, Moon JJ, Lord JD, Yoakim M, Nelson BH, and Neel BG (2000) New role for Shc in activation of the phosphatidylinositol 3-kinase/Akt pathway. Mol Cell Biol 20:7109–7120

Haglund K, Sigismund S, Polo S, Szymkiewicz I, Di Fiore PP, and Dikic I (2003) Multiple monoubiquitination of RTKs is sufficient for their endocytosis and degradation. Nat Cell Biol 5:461–466

Hall A (1998) Rho GTPases and the actin cytoskeleton. Science 279:509–514

Hémar A, Subtil A, Lieb M, Morelon E, Hellio R, and Dautry-Varsat A (1995) Endocytosis of interleukin 2 receptors in human T lymphocytes: distinct intracellular localization and fate of the receptor α, β and γ chains. J Cell Biol 129:55–64

Hicke L, and Riezman H (1996) Ubiquitination of a yeast plasma membrane receptor signals its ligand-stimulated endocytosis. Cell 84:277–287

Hofmann K, and Bucher P (1996) The UBA domain: a sequence motif present in multiple enzyme classes of the ubiquitination pathway. Trends Biochem Sci 21:172–173

Imada K, and Leonard WJ (2000) The Jak-STAT pathway. Mol Immunol 37:1–11

Jiang k, Zhong B, Ritchey C, Gilvary DL, Hong-Geller E, Wei S, and Djeu JY (2003) Regulation of Akt-dependent cell survival by Syk and Rac. Blood 101:236–244

Johannes L, and Lamaze C (2002) Clathrin-dependent or not : is it still the question ? Traffic 3:443–451

Karnitz LM, Burns LA, Sutor SL, Blenis J, and Abraham RT (1995) Interleukin-2 triggers a novel phosphatidylinositol 3-kinase-dependent MEK activation pathway. Mol Cell Biol 15:3049–3057

Katzmann DJ, Babst M, and Emr SD (2001) Ubiquitin-dependent sorting into the multivesicular body pathway requires the function of a conserved endosomal protein sorting complex, ESCRT-I. Cell 106:145–155

Klapisz E, Sorokina I, Lemeer S, Pijnenburg M, Verkleij AJ, and van Bergen en Henegouwen PM (2002) A ubiquitin-interacting motif (UIM) is essential for Eps15 and Eps15R ubiquitination. J Biol Chem 277:30746–30753

Kobayashi N, Kono T, Hatakeyama M, Minami Y, Miyazaki T, Perlmutter RM, and Taniguchi T (1993) Functional coupling of the src-family protein tyrosine kinases p59[fyn] and p53/56[lyn] with the interleukin 2 receptor: Implications for redundancy and pleiotropism in cytokine signal transduction. Proc Natl Acad Sci USA 90:4201–4205

Kohn DB, Sadelain M, and Glorioso JC (2003) Occurrence of leukaemia following gene therapy of X-linked SCID. Nat Rev Cancer 3:477–488

Komada M, and Kitamura N (1995) Growth factor-induced tyrosine phosphorylation of Hrs, a novel 115-kilodalton protein with a structurally conserved putative zinc finger domain. Mol Cell Biol 15:6213–6221

Koyasu S (2003) The role of PI3 K in immune cells. Nat Immunol 4:313–319.

Kurzchalia TV, and Parton RG (1999) Membrane microdomains and caveolae. Curr Opin Cell Biol 11:424–431

Lamaze C, Chuang T-H, Terlecky LJ, Bokoch GM, and Schmid SL (1996) Regulation of receptor-mediated endocytosis by Rho and Rac. Nature 382:177–179

Lamaze C, Dujeancourt A, Baba T, Lo C, Benmerah A, and Dautry-Varsat A (2001) Interleukin 2 receptors and detergent-resistant membrane domains define a clathrin-independent endocytic pathway. Mol Cell 7:661–671

Langdon WY, Hartley JW, Klinken SP, Ruscetti SK, and Morse HC, 3rd (1989) v-cbl, an oncogene from a dual-recombinant murine retrovirus that induces early B-lineage lymphomas. Proc Natl Acad Sci USA 86:1168–1172

Leonard WJ, and Lin J-X (2000) Cytokine receptor signaling pathways. J Allergy Clin Immunol 105:877–888

Leonard WJ (2001) Cytokines and immunodeficiency diseases. Nat Rev Immunol 1:200–208

Lin J-X, and Leonard WJ (2000) The role of Stat5a and Stat5b in signaling by IL-2 family cytokines. Oncogene 19:2566–2576

Lupher ML, Jr., Rao N, Lill NL, Andoniou CE, Miyake S, Clark EA, Druker B, and Band H (1998) Cbl-mediated negative regulation of the Syk tyrosine kinase. A critical role for Cbl phosphotyrosine-binding domain binding to Syk phosphotyrosine 323. J Biol Chem 273:35273–35281.

Marmor MD, and Julius M (2001) Role for lipid rafts in regulating interleukin-2 receptor signaling. Blood 98:1489–1497

Matko J, Bodnar A, Vereb G, Bene L, Vamosi G, Szentesi G, Szöllosi J, Gaspar Jr R, Horejsi V, Waldmann TA, and Damjanovich S (2002) GPI-microdomains (membrane rafts) and signaling of the multi-chain interleukin-2 receptor in human lymphoma/leukemia T cell lines. Eur J Biochem 269:1199–1208

Migone TS, Humbert M, Rascle A, Sanden D, D'Andrea A, and Johnston JA (2001) The deubiquitinating enzyme DUB-2 prolongs cytokine-induced signal transducers and activators of transcription activation and suppresses apoptosis following cytokine withdrawal. Blood 98:1935–1941

Minami Y, Kono T, Miyazaki T, and Taniguchi T (1993) The IL2 receptor complex: its structure, function, and target genes. Annu Rev Immunol 11:245–267

Miyake S, Mullane-Robinson KP, Lill NL, Douillard P, and Band H (1999) Cbl-mediated negative regulation of platelet-derived growth factor receptor-dependent cell proliferation. A critical role for Cbl tyrosine kinase-binding domain. J Biol Chem 274:16619–16628.

Mizuno E, Kawahata K, Kato M, Kitamura N, and Komada M (2003) STAM proteins bind ubiquitinated proteins on the early endosome via the VHS domain and ubiquitin-interacting motif. Mol Biol Cell 14:3675–3689

Molina TJ, Kishihara K, Siderovski DP, Van Ewijk W, Narendran A, Timms E, Wakeham A, Paige CJ, Hartmann K-U, Veillette A, Davidson D, and Mak TW

(1992) Profound block in thymocyte development in mice lacking p56^{lck}. Nature 357:161–164

Morelon E, Dautry-Varsat A, Le Deist F, Fischer A, and de Saint Basile G (1996) T lymphocyte differentiation and proliferation in the absence of the cytoplasmic tail of the common cytokine receptor γ chain in a SCIDX1 patient. Blood 88:1708–1717

Morelon E, and Dautry-Varsat A (1998) Endocytosis of the common cytokine receptor γc chain: identification of sequences involved in internalization and degradation. J Biol Chem 273:22044–22051

Nabi IR, and Le PU (2003) Caveolae/raft-dependent endocytosis. J Cell Biol 161:673–677

Naga Prasad SV, Laporte SA, Chamberlain D, Caron MG, Barak L, and Rockman HA (2002) Phosphoinositide 3-kinase regulates beta2-adrenergic receptor endocytosis by AP-2 recruitment to the receptor/beta-arrestin complex. J Cell Biol 158:563–575.

Nakatsu F, Sakuma M, Matsuo Y, Arase H, Yamasaki S, Nakamura N, Saito T, and Ohno H (2000) A Di-leucine signal in the ubiquitin moiety. Possible involvement in ubiquitination-mediated endocytosis. J Biol Chem 275:26213–26219

Neel BG, Gu H, and Pao L (2003) The 'Shp'ing news: SH2 domain-containing tyrosine phosphatases in cell signaling. Trends Biochem Sci 28:284–293

Nichols BJ (2002) A distinct class of endosome mediates clathrin-independent endocytosis to the Golgi complex. Nat Cell Biol 4:374–378

Odai H, Sasaki K, Iwamatsu A, Hanazono Y, Tanaka T, Mitani K, Yazaki Y, and Hirai H (1995) The proto-oncogene product c-Cbl becomes tyrosine phosphorylated by stimulation with GM-CSF or Epo and constitutively binds to the SH3 domain of Grb2/Ash in human hematopoietic cells. J Biol Chem 270:10800–10805

Pelchen-Matthews A, da Silva RP, Bijlmakers MJ, Signoret N, Gordon S, and Marsh M (1998) Lack of p56lck expression correlates with CD4 endocytosis in primary lymphoid and myeloid cells. Eur J Immunol 28:3639–3647

Pelkmans L, and Helenius A (2003) Insider information : what viruses tell us about endocytosis. Curr Opin Cell Biol 15:414–422

Pitcher C, Honing S, Fingerhut A, Bowers K, and Marsh M (1999) Cluster of differentiation antigen 4 (CD4) endocytosis and adaptor complex binding require activation of the CD4 endocytosis signal by serine phosphorylation. Mol Biol Cell 10:677–691

Polo S, Sigismund S, Faretta M, Guidi M, Capua MR, Bossi G, Chen H, De Camilli P, and Di Fiore PP (2002) A single motif responsible for ubiquitin recognition and monoubiquitination in endocytic proteins. Nature 416:451–455

Raiborg C, Bache KG, Gillooly DJ, Madshus IH, Stang E, and Stenmark H (2002) Hrs sorts ubiquitinated proteins into clathrin-coated microdomains of early endosomes. Nat Cell Biol 4:394–398

Rappoport JZ, Taha BW, and Simon SM (2003) Movement of plasma-membrane-associated clathrin spots along the microtubule cytoskeleton. Traffic 4:460–467

Ravichandran KS, and Burakoff SJ (1994) The adapter protein Shc interacts with the interkeukin-2 (IL-2) receptor upon IL-2 stimulation. J Biol Chem 269:1599–1602

Rocca A, Lamaze C, Subtil A, and Dautry-Varsat A (2001) Involvement of the ubiquitin/proteasome system in sorting of the IL2 receptor β chain to late endocytic compartments. Mol Biol Cell 12:1293–1301

Rodig SJ, Meraz MA, White JM, Lampe PA, Riley JK, Arthur CD, King KL, Sheehan KCF, Yin L, Pennica D, Johnson J, M., and Schreiber RD (1998) Disruption of the *Jak1* gene demonstrates obligatory and nonredundant roles of the jaks in cytokine-induced biologic responses. Cell 93:373–383

Sabharanjak S, Sharma P, Parton RG, and Mayor S (2002) GPI-anchored proteins are delivered to recycling endosomes via a distinct cdc42-regulated, clathrin-independent pinocytic pathway. Dev Cell 2:411–423

Satoh T, Minami Y, Kono T, Yamada K, Kawahara A, Taniguchi T, and Kaziro Y (1992) Interleukin 2-induced activation of ras requires two domains of interleukin 2 receptor β subunit, the essential region for growth stimulation and lck-binding domain. J Biol Chem 267:25423–25427

Schlegel A, and Lisanti MP (2001) Caveolae and their coat proteins, the caveolins : from electron microscopic novelty to biological launching pad. J Cell Physiol 186:329–337

Schoenwaelder SM (2000) The protein tyrosine phosphatase Shp-2 regulates RhoA activity. Curr Biol 10:1523–1526

Shih SC, Katzmann DJ, Schnell JD, Sutanto M, Emr SD, and Hicke L (2002) Epsins and Vps27p/Hrs contain ubiquitin-binding domains that function in receptor endocytosis. Nat Cell Biol 4:389–393

Shih SC, Prag G, Francis SA, Sutanto MA, Hurley JH, and Hicke L (2003) A ubiquitin-binding motif required for intramolecular monoubiquitylation, the CUE domain. EMBO J 22:1273–1281

Simons K, and Ehehalt R (2002) Cholesterol, lipid rafts, and disease. J Clin Invest 110:597–603.

Sorkin A, and Von Zastrow M (2002) Signal transduction and endocytosis: close encounters of many kinds. Nat Rev Mol Cell Biol 3:600–614

Stenmark H, and Aasland R (1999) FYVE-finger proteins–effectors of an inositol lipid. J Cell Sci 112 (Pt 23):4175–4183

Subramaniam PS, and Johnson HM (2002) Lipid microdomains are required sites for the selective endocytosis and nuclear translocation of IFN-γ, its receptor chain IFN-γ receptor-1, and the phosphorylation and nuclear translocation of STAT1α. J Immunol 169:1959–1969

Subtil A, Hémar A, and Dautry-Varsat A (1994) Rapid endocytosis of interleukin 2 receptors when clathrin-coated pit endocytosis is inhibited. J Cell Sci 107:3461–3468

Subtil A, and Dautry-Varsat A (1997) Microtubule depolymerization inhibits clathrin-coated-pit internalization in non-adherent cell lines while interleukin 2 endocytosis is not affected. J Cell Sci 110:2441–2447

Subtil A, Delepierre M, and Dautry-Varsat A (1997) An α-helical signal in the cytosolic domain of the interleukin 2 receptor β chain mediates sorting towards degradation after endocytosis. J Cell Biol 136:583–595

Subtil A, and Dautry-Varsat A (1998) Several weak signals in the cytosolic and transmembrane domains of the interleukin 2 receptor β chain allow for its efficient endocytosis. Eur J Biochem 253:525–530

Subtil A, Rocca A, and Dautry-Varsat A (1998) Molecular characterization of the signal responsible for the targeting of the IL2 receptor β chain toward intracellular degradation. J Biol Chem 273:29424–29429

Takenawa T, and Itoh T (2001) Phosphoinositides, key molecules for regulation of actin cytoskeletal organization and membrane traffic from the plasma membrane. Biochim Biophys Acta 1533:190–206

Tanaka N, Kaneko K, Asao H, Kasai H, Endo Y, Fujita T, Takeshita T, and Sugamura K (1999) Possible involvement of a novel STAM-associated molecule "AMSH" in intracellular signal transduction mediated by cytokines. J Biol Chem 274:19129–19135.

Taniguchi T (1995) Cytokine signaling through nonreceptor protein tyrosine kinases. Science 268:251–255

Thien CB, and Langdon WY (2001) Cbl: many adaptations to regulate protein tyrosine kinases. Nat Rev Mol Cell Biol 2:294–307

Turner M, Mee PJ, Costello PS, Williams O, Price AA, Duddy LP, Furlong MT, Geahlen RL, and Tybulewicz VL (1995) Perinatal lethality and blocked B-cell development in mice lacking the tyrosine kinase Syk. Nature 378:298–302.

van Deurs B, Roepstorff K, Hommelgaard AM, and Sandvig K (2003) Caveolae: Anchored, multifunctional platforms in the lipid ocean. Trends Cell Biol 13:92–100

Vereb G, Matko J, Vamosi G, Ibrahim SM, Magyar E, Varga S, Szöllosi J, Jenei A, Gaspar RJ, Waldmann TA, and Damjanovich S (2000) Cholesterol-dependent clustering of IL-2Rα and its colocalization with HLA and CD48 on T lymphoma cells suggest their functional association with lipid rafts. Proc Natl Acad Sci 97:6013–6018

Waldmann TA (2002) The IL-2/IL-15 receptor systems: Targets for immunotherapy. J Clin Immunol 22:51–56

Waterman H, Levkowitz G, Alroy I, and Yarden Y (1999) The RING finger of c-Cbl mediates desensitization of the epidermal growth factor receptor. J Biol Chem 274:22151–22154

Weissman AM (2001) Themes and variations on ubiquitylation. Nat Rev Mol Cell Biol 2:169–178

Yu A, Olosz F, Choi CY, and Malek TR (2000a) Efficient internalization of IL-2 depends on the distal portion of the cytoplasmic tail of the IL-2R common γ-chain and a lymphoid cell environment. J Immunol 165:2556–2562

Yu CL, Jin YJ, and Burakoff SJ (2000b) Cytosolic tyrosine dephosphorylation of STAT5. Potential role of SHP-2 in STAT5 regulation. J Biol Chem 275:599–604

Zhou YJ, Magnuson KS, Cheng TP, Gadina M, Frucht DM, Galon J, Candotti F, Geahlen RL, Changelian PS, and O'Shea JJ (2000) Hierarchy of protein tyrosine kinases in interleukin-2 (IL-2) signaling: Activation of syk depends on jak3; however, neither syk nor Lck is required for IL-2 mediated STAT activation. Mol Cell Biol 20:4371–4380

Zhu Y (1997) DUB-2 is a member of a novel family of cytokine-inducible deubiquitinating enzymes. J Biol Chem 272:51–57

CTMI (2004) 286:149–185
© Springer-Verlag 2004

Signaling Through Monoubiquitination

S. Sigismund[1] · S. Polo[2] · P. P. Di Fiore (✉)[1, 2, 3]

[1] IFOM, The FIRC Institute for Molecular Oncology, Via Adamello 16,
20139 Milan, Italy
[2] European Institute of Oncology, Via Ripamonti 435, 20141 Milan, Italy
[3] University of Milan, 20122 Milan, Italy
difiore@ifom-firc.it

Abstract Ubiquitination is a post-translational modification in which a small conserved peptide, ubiquitin, is appended to target proteins in the cell, through a series of complex enzymatic reactions. Recently, a particular form of ubiquitination, monoubiquitination, has emerged as a nonproteolytic reversible modification that controls protein function. In this review, we highlight recent findings on monoubiquitination as a signaling-induced modification, controlled, among others, by pathways originating from active receptor tyrosine kinases. Furthermore, we review the major cellular processes controlled by ubiquitin modification, including membrane trafficking, histone function, transcription regulation, DNA repair, and DNA replication.

1
Introduction

Ubiquitination is a post-translational modification in which a small conserved peptide, ubiquitin, is appended to target proteins in the cell, through a series of complex enzymatic reactions. For many years, it has been regarded as a major signal to direct proteins to proteolytic degradation in the 26 S proteasome, thus affecting protein stability and half-life, with profound impacts on cellular homeostasis (Pickart 2000). Indeed, recent studies of the ubiquitin proteome in yeast indicate that a sizable fraction of all protein species are subjected to this regulation (Peng et al. 2003; Hitchcock et al. 2003).

More recently, ubiquitination has emerged as a modifier of protein function as well. A particular form of ubiquitination, monoubiquitination, has been implicated in functions as diverse as regulation of intracellular membrane trafficking, virus budding, and control of transcription and DNA replication (Hicke 2001; Gregory et al. 2003). In addition, monoubiquitination is regulated by signaling events (Di Fiore et al. 2003). The molecular basis of how ubiquitin-based signals are read by the cell is also being elucidated. In summary, ubiquitination is being established as a far-reaching and versatile modification that controls a network of physical and functional interactions with vast ramifications in many cellular processes.

In this review, we initially describe the "components" of the ubiquitin system. We then concentrate on recent findings that establish that monoubiquitination is a signaling-induced modification, controlled, among others, by pathways originating from active receptor tyrosine kinases. Furthermore, we review the major cellular processes controlled by ubiquitin modification, including membrane trafficking, histone function, control of the activation of certain transcription factors, DNA repair, and DNA replication. Finally, we analyze possible models that explain the specificity of ubiquitination reactions, leading to either protein degradation or control of protein function.

2
The Ubiquitin Pathway

2.1
The Ubiquitination Machinery

Ubiquitin (Ub) is a conserved 76-amino acid protein that is covalently conjugated to other proteins through an isopeptide bond between its C-terminal glycine and the ϵ-amino group of lysine residues in substrate proteins (Hershko and Ciechanover 1998). Ubiquitination is a multistep process involving at least three types of enzymes. In the first step, a Ub-activating enzyme (E1) forms a thiol-ester bond between its cysteine located in the active site and the carboxy terminal of Ub, in an ATP-dependent process. In the second step, Ub is transferred to a similar cysteine in the active site of one of the more than 20 known Ub-conjugating (E2) enzymes (Fig. 1a). Finally, an Ub protein ligase (E3) catalyzes the transfer of Ub from the E2 enzyme to the lysine residues on the substrate. Two major families of E3s are known, HECT type and RING type. In HECT-E3-mediated catalysis, Ub is transferred from the E2 to the active-site cysteine of the HECT domain of the E3 ligase, followed by transfer to substrate. In RING-E3-mediated catalysis, Ub is transferred directly from the E2 to the substrate, while the RING-E3 (frequently a multi-subunit complex) functions as an adaptor between the two (Fig. 1a).

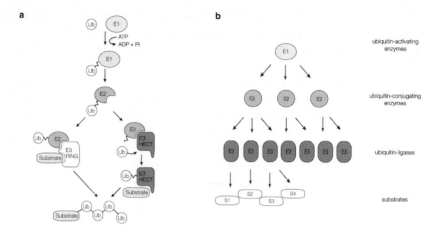

Fig. 1a, b. The ubiquitin pathway. **a** Schematic representation of the ubiquitination process, which involves a cascade of enzymes, E1, E2, and E3 and leads to the ubiquitination of the substrate. **b** A hierarchical view of the enzymes involved in the ubiquitination process is presented, which highlights the increasing complexity of the system (E1-E2-E3) that ensures specificity in substrate recognition

At each step of the ubiquitination process, the complexity of the system increases, and it is ultimately the E3, either alone or in combination with its bound E2, that determines the specificity of substrate recognition. Accordingly, in mammals there are only two E1 isoforms, encoded by a single gene, a few E2 enzymes, and a wide variety of E3 enzymes, probably a few hundreds (Fig. 1b).

Another level of regulation is given by the fact that ubiquitination is a dynamic and reversible process: several deubiquitinating enzymes (DUBs) exist that can reverse this post-translational modification (Wilkinson 2000).

2.2
Different Types of Ubiquitin Signal

Ubiquitin itself can serve as acceptor to form a polyubiquitin chain via several of its seven lysine residues. Thus ubiquitination can occur with different modalities, which have profoundly different effects on the function or the fate of the substrate. Polyubiquitin chains of four or more Ubs, linked through lysine 48, serve as a general device to target proteins for proteolysis by the 26S proteasome (Pickart 2000). Recently, lysine 29-linked Ub chains have also been described and associated with roles in proteasome degradation (Rao and Sastry 2002). Nonproteolytic functions of polyubiquitin have been reported as well, which depend on chains linked through lysine 63. These functions relate mainly to transcription and DNA repair (Gregory et al. 2003; Bach and Ostendorff 2003). Proteins can also be monoubiquitinated, when a single Ub molecule is appended to the substrate, or multiple monoubiquitinated (henceforth also referred to as multiubiquitination), when several lysine residues in the substrate are tagged with single Ub moieties. In general, monoubiquitination serves as a nonproteolytic reversible modification that controls protein function in endocytic trafficking, histone activity, DNA repair, and virus budding (Hicke 2001; Di Fiore et al. 2003; Schnell and Hicke 2003).

3
Modular Ubiquitin Binding Domains

3.1
Ubiquitin-Associated Domains

One way in which cells may interpret Ub signals is exemplified by the existence of small modular protein domains that specifically recognize this modification (Fig. 2). Proteins harboring these modules are globally referred as ubiquitin receptors.

One of these domains, the ubiquitin-associated (UBA) domain, is a short conserved region of ~45 residues, found in many proteins with roles in the Ub proteasome pathway (Hofmann and Bucher 1996) (Fig. 2a). Resolved solution structures of UBA domains revealed a three-helix bundle involved in binding with the Ile-44 hydrophobic surface of Ub (Dieckmann et al. 1998; Mueller and Feigon 2002; Kang et al. 2003). Depending on the protein studied and the conditions used, UBA domains bind to monoubiquitin, polyubiquitin chains, and ubiquitinated proteins (Buchberger 2002). In general, the in vitro data suggest a lower affinity for monoubiquitin than for polyubiquitin. Interestingly, recent in vivo data indicate a specificity of some UBA domains in the recognition of different polyubiquitin lysine linkages (Wilkinson et al. 2001). Indeed, UBA domains of Rad23 and DSK2, two proteins involved in delivering substrate to the proteasome, recognize specifically lysine 29- and lysine 48-linked polyubiquitin chains, two modifications involved in proteolysis, but not lysine 63-linked chains, which have nonproteolytic functions (Rao and Sastry 2000; Ortolan et al. 2000).

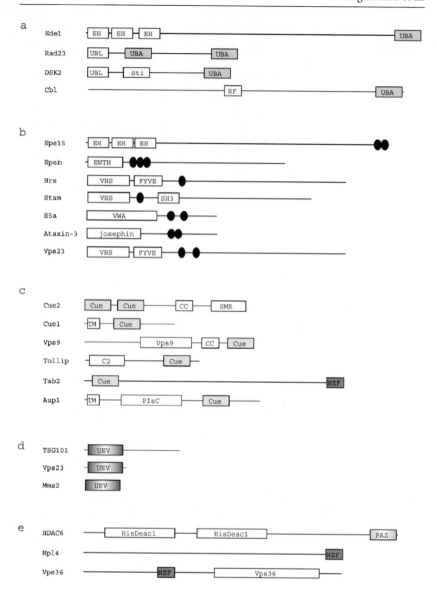

Fig. 2a–e. Ubiquitin-binding modules. The schematic diagram shows the domain architecture of selected Ub-receptors that contain Ub-binding modules: UBA (**a**), UIM (**b**), CUE (**c**), UEV (**d**), and the two Zn finger domains PAZ and NZF (**e**). UIMs are indicated by *black ovals*. Other domains are drawn as *white rectangles* and are labeled as follows: *EH*, Eps15-homology domain; *ENTH*, epsin N-terminal homology domain; *UBL*, ubiquitin-like domain; *FYVE*, FYVE-finger domain; *Josephin*, Josephin

3.2
Ubiquitin-Interacting Motifs

The ubiquitin-interacting motif (UIM) is present in a number of proteins with established or suspected roles in the Ub system (Hofmann and Falquet 2001) (Fig. 2b). It was first identified by database searches for similarity to the 20-amino acid motif of the proteasomal component Rpn10/S5a, which had been previously implicated in polyubiquitin recognition (Pickart 2003). Interestingly, UIMs also occur in a number of proteins involved in endocytosis and vacuolar protein sorting (Fig. 2b). A series of papers demonstrated that UIMs present in this class of proteins, which includes eps15 and eps15R, epsin1 and 2/Ent1 and 2, and Hrs/Hsg/Vps27, are indeed able to bind to Ub (Polo et al. 2002; Raiborg et al. 2002; Bilodeau et al. 2002; Shih et al. 2002; Oldham et al. 2002). More recently, UIMs were also found in a protein involved in polyglutamine neurodegenerative disease, ataxin-3, in which they are involved in binding to polyubiquitinated proteins (Donaldson et al. 2003; Burnett et al. 2003) (Fig. 2b). Finally, UIMs were found in ubiquitin ligases, in deubiquitinating enzymes, and in many other proteins with putative roles in DNA repair and mRNA splicing (Hofmann and Falquet 2001).

The UIM is a very short sequence motif of about 20 residues. The resolved solution structure revealed that it forms a short amphipathic α-helix, in which all of the conserved residues are found exposed on one face and bind to the Ile-44 hydrophobic patch of Ub (Shekhtman and Cowburn 2002; Fisher et al. 2003; Swanson et al. 2003). The affinity of single UIMs for Ub is relatively modest (K_d=0.1–1 mM) (Polo et al. 2002; Raiborg et al.; Fisher et al. 2003). Intriguingly, many UIM-containing proteins harbor multiple copies of the motif, whereas several proteins with a single UIM are found in noncovalent complexes with other UIM-containing partners. In this direction, the UIM of Vps27 crystallized as a tetramer (Fisher et al. 2003). Moreover, mutations within a single UIM, in multi-UIM-containing proteins, produce larger effects than

---

domain involved in Machado-Joseph disease; *RF*, ring finger domain; *SH3*, Src homology domain; *Sti*, repeat domain found in Sti and other proteins; *VHS*, for Vps27, Hrs, Stam domain; *VPS9*, vacuolar protein sorting 9 homology domain (also known as a GEF domain); *VWA*, von Willebrand factor type A domain; *C2*, protein kinase C (PKC) conserved region 2; *CC*, coiled-coil domain; *TM*, transmembrane region; *SMR*, small muts repeated; *PlsC*, phosphate acyltransferase; *Vps36*, Vps36 domain; *HisDeac1*, histone deacetylase domain 1

expected if the motifs were to work in a redundant fashion (Polo et al. 2002; Shih et al. 2002). All these data suggest that a mechanism of high-affinity binding may involve cooperation between multiple UIMs. However, there is also evidence that argues against such a cooperative binding mechanism, at least between tandem UIMs within the same molecule (Swanson et al. 2003).

3.3
The CUE Domain

The CUE domain is a 40 amino acid sequence that was originally identified by database searches because of its similarity to a conserved region of the yeast Cue1 protein (Ponting 2000). Proteins harbouring this domain include endocytic and signaling proteins, such as yeast Vps9p, a guanine nucleotide exchange factor that promotes vesicle fusion with endosomes, mammalian Tollip and TAB2, two proteins involved in interleukin-1 receptor signaling (Donaldson et al. 2003; Shih et al. 2003) (Fig. 2c), AMFR, a cytokine receptor that regulates tumor cell motility and promotes metastasis, and AUP1, a protein involved in integrin signaling. Interestingly, CUE belongs to a class of domains distantly related to UBA, and indeed it has the same structural fold, a three-helix bundle, and interacts with the same hydrophobic surface in the Ub moiety (Kang et al. 2003; Prag et al. 2003). The structure of the CUE-Ub complex reveals that the CUE monomer contains two Ub-binding surfaces on opposite faces that cannot bind simultaneously to a single Ub molecule (Prag et al. 2003). The Vps9 CUE domain crystallized as a dimer and was capable of dimerizing in vivo, as assessed by yeast two-hybrid screening. Dimerization allows two Ub-binding surfaces to contact a single Ub moiety, providing a mechanism for high-affinity binding to monoubiquitin. This is confirmed by the fact that the entire Ub-binding interface formed by the dimer is required for in vivo function (Prag et al. 2003).

3.4
Other Ub-Binding Domains

The ubiquitin E2 enzyme variant (UEV or Ubc-like) domain is related to the catalytic domain found in E2 enzymes but lacks the catalytically important cysteine residue. UEV domains are found in the tumor susceptibility gene protein TSG101/Vps23, which is involved in intracellular trafficking and HIV budding (Bishop et al. 2002), and in Mms2, which has a role in DNA repair (Hoege et al. 2002) (Fig. 2d). In the case of Mms2, the UEV domain associates with a bona fide E2 enzyme (Ubc13) to promote catalysis of Lys-63-linked chains (Hofmann and Pickart 1999). In the case of TSG101/Vps23, the UEV domain instead binds to monoubiquitinated proteins but does not appear to be implicated in catalysis (Katzmann et al. 2001; Garrus et al. 2001). This dual mode of action is reflected also in the fact that the Ub-binding surfaces are different in the two cases, as revealed by the NMR/crystal structures of the two UEV domains (Pornillos et al. 2002; VanDemark et al. 2001; McKenna et al. 2003).

Two zinc finger domains are known to interact with Ub. The first one, named polyubiquitin-associated zinc finger (PAZ) domain, is present in the microtubule histone deacetylase 6 (HDAC6) and is similar to other zinc finger domains present in several Ub-specific proteases (Seigneurin-Berny et al. 2001) (Fig. 2e). It has been shown to bind specifically to polyubiquitin and not to monoubiquitin, both in two-hybrid screenings and in in vitro binding assays (Hook et al. 2002). The second domain is the so-called "novel Zn finger" (NZF) domain. It has been identified in proteins involved in membrane fusion and trafficking, such as Ufd1-Npl4, an adaptor that mediates diverse ubiquitin-dependent function of the p97/CDC48p ATPase, and Vps36, which is involved in vacuolar sorting of ubiquitinated protein (Meyer et al. 2002) (Fig. 2e). The NMR structure shows that the NZF motif is structurally different from UBA, UIM, and CUE domains, consisting primarily of β-strands. Nevertheless, as in the case of the other domains, it binds to the Ile-44 hydrophobic patch on the Ub molecule (Wang et al. 2003).

4
Monoubiquitination as a Signaling-Inducible Post-translational Modification: The Case of Endocytosis

4.1
Multiple Monoubiquitination of RTKs Is Induced by Growth Factors

Ligand-induced ubiquitination of several plasma membrane receptors, including numerous receptor tyrosine kinases (RTKs), has been implicated in the regulation of their internalization and endocytosis (Thien et al. 2001; Dikic et al. 2003; Levkowitz et al. 1998; Miyake et al. 1998; Lee et al. 1999; Taher et al. 2002; Terrell et al. 1998; Shih et al. 2000; Mori et al. 1993). The first evidence that monoubiquitin, and not Ub chains, controls these processes came from studies of Ste2p, a pheromone G protein-coupled receptor in *Saccaromyces cerevisiae* (Terrell et al. 1998). Ste2p internalization and degradation into the yeast vacuole, an equivalent of the mammalian lysosome, is dependent on the Ub acceptor lysine residues in its cytoplasmic domain (Terrell et al. 1998). Importantly, a Ste2p-Ub chimera, in which the cytoplasmic sequence of Ste2p is replaced by a single Ub, results in a chimeric protein that is rapidly internalized and degraded in the vacuole (Shih et al. 2000). More recent studies in mammalian cells have shown that chimeras consisting of monoubiquitin fused to the cytoplasmic regions of the invariant chain of the interleukin-2 receptor α-chain (Nakatsu et al. 2000) or epidermal growth factor receptor (EGFR) can be efficiently downregulated (Haglund et al. 2003; Mosesson et al. 2003). These receptors are constitutively internalized from the cell surface and targeted to the late endosomal/lysosomal compartment (Haglund et al. 2003). In the same studies, it was shown that multiple monoubiquitination, but not formation of Ub chains, is associated with ligand-induced ubiquitination of EGFR and platelet-derived growth factor receptors (PGDFR) (Haglund et al. 2003; Mochida et al. 2002). These findings have provided a molecular explanation of why activated RTKs, which were long thought to be polyubiquitinated, do not undergo proteasomal degradation, but rather follow a completely different route, being degraded in the lysosome.

As discussed more extensively in the next sections, ubiquitination of RTKs seems to act as a critical gating signal in the endosome, by targeting receptors toward the lysosome, whereas it appears to be sufficient but not strictly necessary for receptor internalization (Duan et al. 2003; Wang et al. 2002; Jiang and Sorkin 2003). This could be explained by the presence of multiple internalization pathways at the cell surface, as compared with a more unique role of Ub in endosomal sorting pathways. In accordance with this explanation, the rate of internalization of an EGFR-Ub chimera was lower than that of the wild-type EGFR (Haglund et al. 2003) pointing to the presence of redundant pathways. Such pathways include those based on dileucine and tyrosine-based endocytic motifs in the EGF receptor or those relying on recruitment of the CIN85/endophilin complex, and they act in concert with Ub-dependent signals, at the early steps of receptor internalization (Soubeyran et al. 2002; Petrelli et al. 2002; Sorkin 2001; Brett et al. 2002).

4.2
Accessory Endocytic Proteins Are Monoubiquitinated following RTK Activation

In addition to activated RTKs, receptor-associated proteins may also be ubiquitinated, thus amplifying signals in the Ub network. In some cases, for example, the growth hormone receptor, endocytosis and endosomal sorting do not require receptor ubiquitination but still depend on a functional Ub machinery (Strous et al. 1996; Strous and Gent 2002). In these cases, monoubiquitinated receptor-associated endocytic proteins might be responsible for sorting of the receptors along the endocytic pathway. Indeed, several proteins acting at different steps of the endocytic route are monoubiquitinated following growth factor stimulation (Polo et al. 2002; Shih et al. 2002; Klapisz et al. 2002; van Delft et al. 1997). Among them, eps15 and epsin are involved at early stages of internalization (Brett et al. 2002; Salcini et al. 1999; Chen et al. 1998), where ubiquitinated receptors are recruited into primary endocytic vesicles. Other monoubiquitinated proteins, such as Hrs, function at a later step in the endocytic route, at the endosomal level (Raiborg et al. 2002; Katzmann et al. 2002), where ubiquitinated receptors are sorted to different destinations, either lysosomal degradation or recycling to the plasma membrane. Another example is provided by the adaptor protein CIN85, which functions in EGFR endocytosis (Soubeyran et al. 2002) and is monoubiquitinated by the E3 ligase Cbl following ligand stimulation. Importantly, Cbl is also ubiquitinated in the complex with activated receptors and with monoubiquitinated CIN85 (Wang et al. 1999; Haglund et al. 2002). Because CIN85 tends to form oligomers, it can potentially cluster EGFR/Cbl ubiquitinated complexes (Dikic 2002; Kowanetz et al. 2003). Thus large complexes containing multiple monoubiquitinated proteins could form that traffic throughout the endocytic route, and Ub appears to be one of the major inducible transport signals recognized by the endocytic machinery.

5
Molecular Mechanisms Linking Activated RTKs to the Ubiquitination Machinery: The Role of Cbl

5.1
Cbl as an E3 Ubiquitin Ligase

Cbl is the major E3 ligase involved in RTK ubiquitination on signaling, and thus it plays a pivotal role in regulating receptor internalization, trafficking, and degradation. Following RTK activation, Cbl is recruited to a specific phosphorylated tyrosine residue in the receptor tail (Y1045 in the EGFR) via a direct interaction mediated by the SH2-like domain, contained in Cbl (Levkowitz et al. 1999). Cbl could also bind to RTKs indirectly, through interaction with the Grb2 adaptor protein (Wong et al. 2002; Waterman et al. 2002; Jiang et al. 2003). As a consequence of this physical interaction, Cbl multiubiquitinates the activated receptor (Stang et al. 2000) (Fig. 3). After internalization, Cbl remains associated with RTKs in early and late endosomes. This persistent association might enable Cbl to progressively monoubiquitinate receptors at multiple sites, thus controlling receptor sorting for degradation into the lysosome (de Melker et al. 2001) (Fig. 3).

Cbl is a member of a protein family that is structurally and functionally conserved in multicellular organisms. The E3 Ub ligase activity resides in its RING finger domain. Indeed, overexpression of Cbl enhances ubiquitination and degradation of EGF, PDGF, and CSF-1 receptors (Levkowitz et al. 1998; Miyake et al. 1998; Lee et al. 1999), whereas Cbl mutants, carrying mutations at the level of the RING finger domain, block receptor ubiquitination and degradation by shunting endocytosed receptors from the endosome to the recycling pathway (Levkowitz et al. 1998). Cbl can also mediate EGF-induced monoubiquitination of CIN85, and this requires an intact RING finger domain and a CIN85-binding motif in the C-terminal portion of Cbl (Haglund et al. 2002).

There is also evidence that Cbl functionally interacts with other E3 ligases, leading to a compartment-specific regulation of various signaling pathways. Accordingly, association between Cbl and AIP4, a HECT-type E3 ligase, has been shown also to be important for EGFR downregulation (Courbard et al. 2002). In addition, after immunoglobulin engagement and activation of the high-affinity receptor for IgE, Cbl and Nedd4, another member of the HECT-type E3 family, copartition into lipid rafts, where they may ubiquitinate components of receptor complexes, regulating IgE-triggered signaling occurring in rafts (Lafont and Simons 2001). Recently, Nedd4 was shown to polyubiquitinate Cbl, an event that leads to proteasomal degradation of the latter (Magnifico et al. 2003) (Fig. 3). This is particularly interesting in light of the fact that Nedd4 is probably also activated, like Cbl, by RTKs, because it is responsible for monoubiquitination of eps15 and Hrs following EGFR stimulation (Polo et al. 2002; Katz et al. 2002). It is not clear how EGFR activates Nedd4, because, at variance with what has been shown for Cbl, no interaction between EGFR and Nedd4 can be detected. In this case, it is possible that EGFR-induced downstream events, for instance, serine/threo-

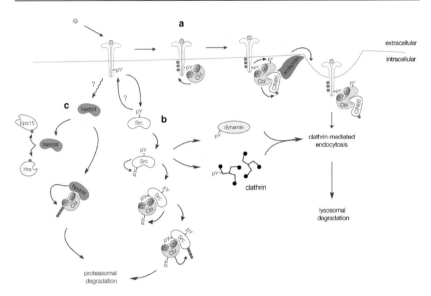

Fig. 3a–c. The Cbl-based signaling network. **a** Modalities of Cbl-mediated multiubiquitination and internalization of the receptor. Following ligand induction, Cbl is recruited to the phosphorylated receptor tail via its SH2-like domain and multiubiquitinates the receptor. Then, Cbl becomes phosphorylated and binds to CIN85, which
is constitutively complexed with endophilin. In this way, endophilin is recruited to
the membrane and can induce membrane curvature, thereby facilitating the internalization step. In addition, CIN85 is monoubiquitinated by Cbl. **b** Mechanisms of
Src regulation by Cbl. Src becomes phosphorylated following RTK activation and, in
turn, is responsible for some phosphorylation events in the receptor tail. Activated
Src is involved in phosphorylation of dynamin and clathrin, which contributes to
the endocytic process. Once phosphorylated, Src binds to Cbl in two ways: via its
SH3 domain (to the proline-rich region of Cbl), and via its phosphotyrosine (pY) (to
the SH2 domain of Cbl). This leads to Cbl-mediated ubiquitination and degradation
of Src. **c** Cooperation between Cbl and Nedd4. Following EGF stimulation, Nedd4 is
activated via an unknown mechanism, possibly involving phosphorylation, and then
is able to monoubiquitinate eps15 and Hrs and to polyubiquitinate Cbl, leading to
its proteasomal degradation. In all panels ubiquitin is represented by a *gray circle*

nine phosphorylation, might modulate the catalytic activity of Nedd4.
Accordingly, phosphorylation on serine residues modulates Nedd4 activity on another of its substrates, the epithelial Na^+ channel (ENaC) (Snyder et al. 2002; Debonneville et al. 2001). Whatever the case, a complex
regulatory interplay between Cbl and HECT-type E3 ligases seems to exist, whose equilibrium might be very relevant to endocytosis and sorting.

5.2
Cbl as a Multifunctional Adaptor Molecule

Recent evidence indicates that Cbl regulates RTK internalization also via pathways that are functionally distinct from its ligase activity and dependent on its protein-protein interaction abilities. Cbl interacts with more than 40 proteins, many of which are implicated in the control of receptor trafficking along the endocytic route, thus positioning Cbl as a link between RTKs and the endocytic regulatory network (Fig. 3). Moreover, Cbl is phosphorylated following numerous external and oncogenic signals, and its phosphorylation was shown to mediate association with several intracellular signaling partners, thus connecting the molecular machinery of endocytosis to that of signal transduction. One well-characterized partner of Cbl is the Src kinase, a major player in receptor endocytosis and signaling. Src binds, phosphorylates and activates dynamin (Ahn et al. 2002) and phosphorylates the heavy chain of clathrin, which then redistributes to the cell periphery and enhances endocytosis (Wilde et al. 1999). Src is directly activated by signaling-induced receptors and subsequently can be switched off by Cbl with different mechanisms. It is clear that Cbl negatively regulates Src activity, working as an SH2-like adaptor (as in the case of integrin signaling, where it binds and inhibits autophosphorylated Src; Sanjay et al. 2001) or as an E3 ligase promoting ubiquitination and degradation of active Src (as in the case of EGFR signaling; Andoniou et al. 2000) (Fig. 3).

Cbl could also regulate RTK internalization by binding to the adaptor protein CIN85 (Soubeyran et al. 2002; Petrelli et al. 2002). After growth factor stimulation, CIN85 is rapidly recruited to Cbl-RTKs complexes at the plasma membrane (Soubeyran et al. 2002; Petrelli et al. 2002; Kirsch et al. 2001; Watanabe et al. 2000). As a consequence, endophilins, which are stably associated with CIN85, are positioned in close proximity to internalizing receptors and can possibly induce negative curvature and invagination of the plasma membrane during the initial steps of the internalization process (Schmidt et al. 1999; Farsad et al. 2001; Ringstad et al. 1999) (Fig. 3). This appears to be a general mechanism involved in internalization of RTKs, including EGFR, PDGFR, c-Met, and c-Kit (Soubeyran et al. 2002; Petrelli et al. 2002; Szymkiewicz et al. 2002). The CIN85-Cbl interaction is also likely to be involved in postinternalization processes, such as receptor trafficking and degradation (Soubeyran et al. 2002; Petrelli et al. 2002; Szymkiewicz et al. 2002), as both CIN85 and Cbl cotraffic with activated RTKs all along the endocytic route and are targeted for common degradation into the lysosome (Haglund et al.

2002) (Fig. 3). Finally, CIN85 might also regulate the process of cargo delivery through regulation of actin dynamics, as it binds Cbl-cargo complexes and components of the actin cytoskeleton (Hutchings et al. 2003).

5.3
Deregulation of Cbl and Neoplastic Growth

Given the centrality of Cbl in the process of receptor internalization and degradation, which in turn limits mitogenic responses, it is not surprising that Cbl can be easily activated as an oncogene. This is the result of deletions or mutations that perturb the ability of Cbl to downregulate RTKs. The oncogenic v-Cbl protein, a truncated form of Cbl containing only the N-terminal portion, associates with RTKs but cannot ubiquitinate the receptors (Thien et al. 2001; Levkowitz et al. 1998; Andoniou et al. 1994). Thus v-Cbl works in a dominant-negative fashion by competing with the endogenous wild-type protein for binding sites on activated RTKs, thereby preventing Cbl-mediated downmodulation and contributing to enhance signaling and oncogenic transformation. Similarly, other transforming forms of Cbl bear deletions or mutations within the RING finger and/or the preceding linker region, as in the case of the naturally occurring oncogenic mutant, 70Z-Cbl (Andoniou et al. 1994). From these findings it is clear that uncoupling Cbl from RTKs results in defective downregulation of receptor activity and in oncogenic transformation. Accordingly, numerous oncogenic RTKs were found to be defective in Cbl-mediated downregulation, such in the case of oncogenic forms of EGFR (Shu et al. 1991; Ekstrand et al. 1992), HGFR (Peschard et al. 2001; Mancini et al. 2002), and CSF-1 receptor (Mancini et al. 2002; Ridge et al. 1990; Baker et al. 1988).

6
Ubiquitin-Mediated Signaling in Membrane Trafficking

6.1
The Dual Function of UIM/CUE Domains as a Molecular Basis for a Network of Ubiquitin-Mediated Interactions

As mentioned above, monoubiquitin is a regulated signal for membrane protein trafficking, recognized by endocytic Ub-binding proteins. A frequent feature of these endocytic proteins is the presence of both Ub-binding domains and monoubiquitination on the same molecule (Polo et al. 2002; Shih et al. 2002; Oldham et al. 2002; Shih et al. 2003; Klapisz et al. 2002). These two molecular functions are intimately linked, as it was shown that UIMs and CUEs, in addition to binding to Ub, are also indispensable for monoubiquitination of the proteins in which they are contained (Polo et al. 2002; Shih et al. 2003). The dual function of these domains might determine extensive networking abilities, in that proteins that are monoubiquitinated (by virtue of the presence of UIM/CUE) can also establish inter- and intramolecular interactions with other Ub- or UIM/CUE-containing proteins, thus generating a network of Ub-mediated interactions, which can influence many aspects of cellular physiology (Di Fiore, et al. 2003). Interestingly, several Ub receptors are monoubiquitinated in a signaling-dependent manner (Polo et al. 2002; Klapisz et al. 2002; van Delft et al. 1997; Haglund et al. 2002). Thus they could contribute to events leading to intracellular signal transduction and/or to endosomal sorting. The molecular connections downstream of receptor ubiquitination are now starting to be elucidated by studies showing that intact Ub-binding modules, in a series of Ub receptors, are required at different steps of the endocytic route. These findings are discussed in the following sections.

6.2
Ubiquitin Receptors at the Initial Steps of Internalization

As previously discussed, Ub appears to be the most common internalization signal employed by *S. cerevisiae* (Hicke 2001). Shih and coworkers have recently demonstrated that the Ub receptors Ent1p/Ent2p and Ede1p (the homologs of human epsins and eps15, respectively) are required for the internalization of the pheromone receptor Ste2p into vesi-

Fig. 4A–D. Ubiquitin receptors in membrane trafficking. **A** Involvement of eps15 and epsin at the initial step of the internalization process. eps15 and epsin bind to the ubiquitinated receptor, through their UIMs, and possibly recruit AP2 and clathrin to the activated receptor, because of their ability to bind to these endocytic proteins. **B** Possible regulation of endosome fusion by Rabex5. Rabex5 shifts from an inactive/close conformation to an active/open conformation on its interaction, mediated by the CUE domain, with the ubiquitinated receptor. This allows Rabex5 to exert its GEF activity on Rab5, leading to endosome fusion. This model is proposed for mammalian Rab5 and Rabex5 in analogy to what has been reported in yeast for Vps9 and Vps21 (see main text for details). **C** Recognition of ubiquitinated cargo at the endosomal level by an Hrs-eps15-STAM complex. **D** Sorting of the ubiquitinated cargo to

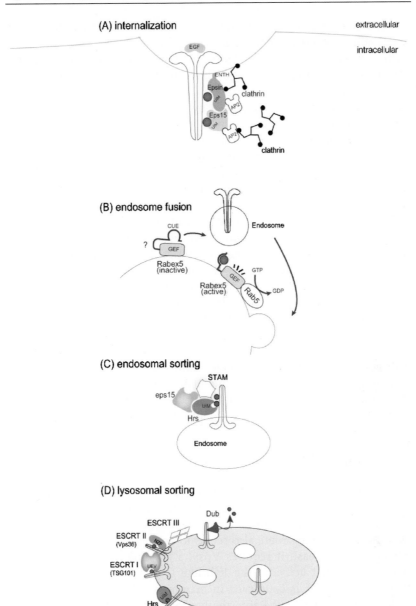

(A) internalization

(B) endosome fusion

(C) endosomal sorting

(D) lysosomal sorting

the lysosome, by the sequential action of ESCRT complexes that select the ubiquitinated cargo on MVBs. After a deubiquitination step, the cargo is sequestered into the inner vesicles of MVBs and sorted for degradation into the lysosome. In all panels ubiquitin is represented by a *gray circle*

cles at the plasma membrane. Moreover, at least in the case of Ents, their function is dependent on intact UIMs (Shih et al. 2002). Albeit not demonstrated yet, it is very likely that Ent1p/Ent2p and Ede1p represent Ub receptors for ubiquitinated Ste2p. This is particularly interesting in light of findings that a chimeric Ste2p-Ub molecule, in which all Ste2p cytoplasmic tail sequences are replaced by a single Ub moiety, can be efficiently internalized (Shih et al. 2000).

In mammalian cells, eps15 and epsins are the likely candidates to act as plasma membrane Ub receptors that couple monoubiquitin-containing RTKs with the endocytic machinery (Di Fiore et al. 2003). They could directly bind to monoubiquitinated receptors via their UIMs and, at the same time, interact with the clathrin adaptor protein AP-2 through their DPF and DPW motifs, recruiting the downstream endocytic machinery (Brett et al. 2002; Salcini et al. 1999; Drake et al. 2000) (Fig. 4). In support of this model, a chimeric receptor, whose internalization is mediated solely by the Ub signal, is constitutively internalized (Haglund et al. 2003) through its interaction with the UIM-containing proteins eps15 and epsin (S. Sigismund, S. Polo, P.P. Di Fiore, unpublished data). This is interesting in light of findings that AP-2, the major adaptor for clathrin, has been shown to be dispensable for endocytosis of EGF receptors (Hinrichsen et al. 2003; Motley et al. 2003). In this scenario, ubiquitination might provide additional and /or redundant levels of action, by recruiting Ub-dependent machinery to internalize receptors. Thus Ub adaptors can work in parallel or in concert with the well-established endocytic machinery to optimize the internalization step.

6.3
Ubiquitin Receptors in Endosome Fusion

After pinching off from the plasma membrane, coated vesicles undergo clathrin shedding and fuse with an acceptor compartment forming the early endosomes, where the second major sorting event occurs. This step of the trafficking route also seems to be controlled by Ub-mediated interactions. In yeast, it requires Vps9, a guanine nucleotide exchange factor (GEF) that activates the Rab-like GTP-ase Vps21 (Hama et al. 1999). This system is conserved in mammals, where Rabex-5 (the homolog of Vps9) activates Rab5 (the homolog of Vps21) (Horiuchi et al. 1997). Rab5 has in turn been shown to regulate the trafficking of a number of receptors (Volpicelli et al. 2001; Barbieri et al. 2000; Seachrist et al. 2002). Both Vps9 and Rabex5 promote membrane fusion at the level of the endosomes and possess a CUE domain in their C-termini. Studies of the mode of action of the CUE domain of Vps9 revealed that it inhibits *in cis* the GEF activity toward Vps21. Moreover, the CUE domain of Vps9 interacts physically and genetically with Ub, and this interaction is critical to unmask its enzymatic activity and for vacuolar delivery of ubiquitinated cargoes (Donaldson et al. 2003). Thus a model can be envisioned in which the interaction of the CUE of Vps9 with ubiquitinated receptor tails relieves the self-inhibitory conformation of Vps9, allowing activation of Vps21 and endosomal membrane fusion (Fig. 4). Finally, the CUE domain is absolutely required for monoubiquitination of Vps9, which is executed by Rsp5, the yeast homolog of Nedd4 (Shih et al. 2003). This suggests the intriguing possibility that the self-inhibited conformation of Vps9 is dictated by an intramolecular interaction between monoubiquitin and CUE, *in cis* on the Vps9 molecule.

6.4
Receptor Downregulation and Multivesicular Body Sorting

Although there is still debate as to whether trafficking from the early endosomes to the next compartment in the endocytic route involves vesicular transport or maturation, the cargo proteins proceed into a compartment called the multivesicular body (MVB), characterized by multiple internal vesicles and low luminal pH. At this step, recycling receptors are redirected to the plasma membrane, while ubiquitinated receptors are prevented from recycling by becoming sequestered inside the MVB (Katzmann et al. 2002). The conservation of this pathway from yeast to human highlights the importance of this transport route in all eukaryotic cells. Recent findings indicate that the UIM-containing proteins Hrs, eps15, and signal-transducing adaptor molecule (STAM) form a multivalent Ub-binding complex on early endosomes, sorting endocytic cargoes into the MVB pathway (Bache et al. 2003) (Fig. 4). Hrs seems to be the key player at this step: KO mice, as well as yeast defective strains, showed enlarged endosomes and impairment of the delivery of cargoes to the lysosome/vacuole (Shih et al. 2002; Komada and Soriano 1999; Piper et al. 1995). Strikingly, the UIM of Hrs has been recently shown to be absolutely required for the recognition of ubiquitinated cargoes at this sorting step (Raiborg et al. 2002; Bilodeau et al. 2002; Shih et al. 2002; Bishop et al. 2002).

At the outer membrane of the MVB an internalization-like step takes place, leading to inward budding of small cargo-containing vesicles that will eventually merge with the lysosome and be degraded (Katzmann et al. 2002). At this step tumor susceptibility gene product 101 (TSG101)

(Bishop et al. 2002; Garrus et al. 2001), a component of the endosomal sorting complex required for transport ESCRT-I complex comes into play (Katzmann et al. 2001). TSG101 contains a UEV/UBC domain, which interacts with Ub and selects ubiquitinated cargoes that should be sorted into the inner vesicles of the MVB and further degraded into the lysosome (Bishop et al. 2002; Katzmann et al. 2001; Katzmann et al. 2002) (Fig. 4). In support of the importance of this regulation, EGFR downregulation is impaired in mouse fibroblasts lacking TSG101, and this leads to tumors in nude mice (Li and Cohen 1996).

Other complexes are sequentially required for the sorting of cargoes into invaginating vesicles during MVB formation: ESCRTII (which is composed of Vps22, Vps25, and Vps36) (Babst et al. 2002) seems to direct the ESCRTIII complex to the appropriate endosomal membrane, whereas ESCRTIII (which is composed of Vps20, Snf7, Vps2, and Vps24) (Babst et al. 2003) seems to have a role in the concentration of the cargoes and in the recruitment of the Doa4 protein. This deubiquitinating enzyme acts at the latest step, to recover Ub from membrane cargoes in route to the vacuole and to facilitate Ub recycling (Katzmann et al. 2002) (Fig. 4).

In conclusion, Ub appears to be the critical signal that sorts receptors for degradation in the lysosome in order to prevent their recycling and to ensure termination of signals.

7
Ubiquitin-Mediated Signaling in Transcription and DNA Repair

7.1
Histone Regulation by Monoubiquitin:
Cross-Talk Between Ubiquitination and Methylation

In eukaryotes, transcription of protein-encoding genes is regulated by chromatin structure and by a large set of proteins including transcription factors, coactivators/corepressors, and general initiation and elongation factors, all of which can be influenced by signaling pathways (Naar et al. 2001). Several types of protein modifications, including phosphorylation, methylation, acetylation, and more recently, ubiquitination, have been associated with the regulation of gene expression. In recent years, important connections between signaling, ubiquitination, chromatin structure, and transcriptional control have emerged. In yeast, the histone H2B C-terminal tail was shown to be monoubiquitinated in vivo by the E2 enzyme Rad6/Ubc2 and by the RING-type E3 ligase Bre1 (Robzyk et al. 2000; Hwang et al. 2003; Wood et al. 2003). This monoubiquitination event, which does not lead to degradation of H2B, was demonstrated to be crucial for mitotic and meiotic growth (Robzyk et al. 2000). Similarly, a subunit of the transcription factor TFIID was shown to monoubiquitinate histone H1 in *Drosophila*, and this modification is essential for the correct sequential expression of certain genes during development (Pham and Sauer 2000).

The "histone-code" hypothesis proposes that post-translational modifications in histone tails are "read" by other histones and/or proteins and are translated into silencing or activation of gene transcription (Bach and Ostendorff 2003). Recent research on the role of monoubiquitination in the context of other post-translational modifications supports this hypothesis. Accordingly, Rad6-mediated monoubiquitination of histone H2B has been shown to be a prerequisite for H3 methylation on K4 and K69, key events in the regulation of gene expression (Dover et al. 2002; Briggs et al. 2002). Mutations of the lysines that are acceptor sites of monoubiquitination in H2B abolish gene silencing at telomeric regions caused by methylation. These findings evidence a functional link between ubiquitination, methylation, and gene silencing (Dover et al. 2002; Sun and Allis 2002) and establish monoubiquitination as a powerful upstream regulator of histone function.

7.2
Signal-induced Ubiquitination of IκB Kinase β: Cross-Talk Between Phosphorylation and Ubiquitination

The initiation of the genetic programs for inflammation and immunity involves nuclear translocation of the transcription factor NF-κB (Li and Verma 2002). This signal-dependent process is controlled in part by the β catalytic subunit of IκB kinase (IKKβ), which targets IκBα and other cytoplasmic inhibitors of NF-κB for proteolytic destruction (Zandi and Karin 1999). The catalytic activity of IKKβ is stimulated by pathological and physiological inducers of NF-κB, such as Tax oncoprotein (Sun and Ballard 1999) and proinflammatory cytokines (Delhase et al. 1999). Following such signaling events, IKKβ becomes phosphorylated and monoubiquitinated (Delhase et al. 1999; Carter et al. 2001; Carter et al. 2003). Loss-of-function mutations that block phosphorylation of IKKβ prevent its ubiquitination (Carter et al. 2003). Therefore, phosphorylation seems to serve as a substrate recognition motif, allowing the ubiquitination machinery to dock with and monoubiquitinate IKKβ. In ad-

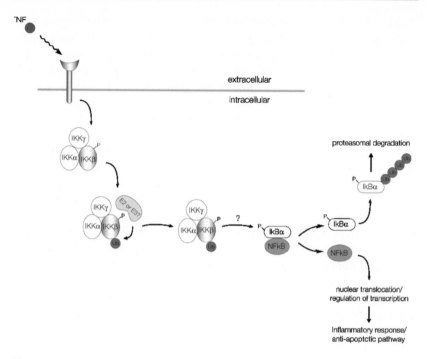

Fig. 5. Monoubiquitination of IKKβ. Following TNF stimulation, IKKβ becomes phosphorylated, allowing the recruitment of the Ub machinery, which, in turn, monoubiquitinates IKKβ. These two modifications seem to be required for the catalytic activity of IKKβ toward IkBα, the NFκB inhibitor. Once phosphorylated by IKKβ, IκBα is targeted for degradation, allowing NFκB translocation into the nucleus and activation of transcription

dition, gain-of-function mutants are constitutively monoubiquitinated, projecting an important role for ubiquitin in the modulation of IKKβ function (Carter et al. 2003) (Fig. 5).

7.3
Monoubiquitination and K63-Linked Polyubiquitination in DNA Repair

During replication, DNA lesions can block progression of the DNA polymerase, necessitating DNA repair, a process that is highly conserved from yeast to human. Genetic studies in yeast have identified two mechanisms that allow replication to bypass the DNA lesion, both of which are dependent on the E2 enzyme Rad6. One mechanism, the "error-free" mechanism, uses the undamaged sister duplex at the replication forks as a template; the other, the "error-prone" mechanism, utilizes trans-lesion polymerases that add correct or incorrect nucleotides across the damaged site (Bach and Ostendorff 2003). Monoubiquitination and lysine 63-linked polyubiquitination are emerging as signals involved in these two pathways. In addition, a small-ubiquitin-related modifier, SUMO (Melchior 2000), uses a similar conjugation system that sometimes counteracts the effects of ubiquitination. Indeed, Ub and SUMO compete for modification of the proliferating cell nuclear antigen (PCNA), an essential processivity factor for DNA replication and repair (Hoege et al. 2002). PCNA was shown to be modified by Rad6-mediated sumoylation, monoubiquitination, and K63-linked polyubiquitination (Hoege et al. 2002). All three modifications affect the same lysine residue (conserved from yeast to human) in PCNA, suggesting that they label PCNA for alternative functions. Accordingly, it was shown that the SUMO modification is involved in normal DNA replication during S phase, whereas ubiquitination is clearly linked to DNA damage and to the Rad6-mediated repair pathway (Hoege et al. 2002). In particular, K63-linked polyubiquitination seems to be involved in "error-free" DNA repair whereas monoubiquitination seems to act in the "error-prone" pathway, by promoting trans-lesion DNA synthesis (Stelter and Ulrich 2003) (Fig. 6a).

At the molecular level, following DNA damage, Rad6 appears to monoubiquitinate PCNA. Subsequently, Ubc13-Mms2, a UEV/E2 complex, is recruited, which catalyzes the formation of K63-linked Ub chains onto monoubiquitinated PCNA (Hoege et al. 2002) (Fig. 6a). Finally, as both sumoylation and ubiquitination are reversible processes (Hershko and Ciechanover 1998; Melchior 2000; Muller et al. 2001), a sequential cycle of these two modifications for substrates can be envisioned as a possible regulatory mechanism.

7.4
Monoubiquitin Signal following DNA Damage and During DNA Replication: Fanconi Anemia

In response to genotoxic agents (i.e., ionizing radiation, cross-linking agents) eukaryotic cells mount a protective response to avoid DNA damage and subsequent mutations. First, checkpoint pathways are activated, leading to cell cycle arrest, and then DNA repair pathways are induced and double strand breaks are corrected (Nyberg et al. 2002). Failure to target damage response proteins to DNA repair foci results in the accumulation of excessive mutations, genomic instability, and cancer. Genet-a

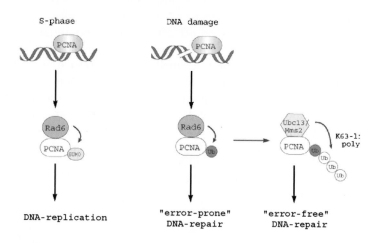

b

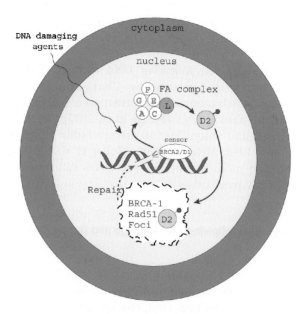

Fig. 6a, b. Ubiquitination and DNA repair. **a** Mechanisms of regulation of PCNA. During normal S phase, PCNA is sumoylated by Rad6 and promotes DNA-replication. Following DNA-damage, PCNA is monoubiquitinated by Rad6 and promotes "error-prone" DNA repair. Alternatively, monoubiquitinated PCNA could be recruited by Ubc13/Mms2, which targets its polyubiquitination through lysine 63, a process

ic and biochemical studies of Fanconi anemia (FA) uncovered a crucial role for monoubiquitination in this response.

Fanconi anemia is an autosomal recessive cancer susceptibility syndrome characterized by multiple congenital anomalies, bone marrow failure, and cellular sensitivity to mitomycin C (MMC) (D'Andrea and Grompe 2003; Taniguchi and Dandrea 2002). Several FA complementation groups, which identify distinct molecular defects, have been identified so far, as assessed by somatic cell fusion analysis of cells derived from patients with the disease (Strathdee et al. 1992; Lo Ten Foe et al. 1996; de Winter et al. 2001; de Winter et al. 2000; de Winter et al. 1998). Eight of the FA genes, including genes for FANCA, FANCC, FANCD1, FANCD2, FANCE, FANCF, FANCG, and FANCL, have been cloned. It is now known that five proteins (FANCA, FANCC, FANCE, FANCF, and FANCG) are assembled in a multimolecular complex (FA complex) that is required for the monoubiquitination of the FANCD2 protein, which occurs after DNA damage and leads to FANCD2 recruitment to BRCA1-containing nuclear foci (Taniguchi and Dandrea 2002; Taniguchi et al. 2002; Garcia-Higuera et al. 1999) (Fig. 6b). Of note, monoubiquitination of FANCD2, mediated by the FA complex, is also a S phase-regulated event during normal cell cycle progression (Taniguchi et al. 2002). In S phase, monoubiquitinated FANCD2 is targeted to BRCA1- and RAD51-containing nuclear foci, where it seems to participate in homologous recombination repair (Taniguchi et al. 2002; Meetei et al. 2003). Disruption of the FA pathway results in the absence of FANCD2-containing nuclear foci, leading to the cellular and clinical abnormalities of FA.

Monoubiquitination appears to require both an intact FA complex and the BRCA1 protein. Surprisingly, the FA complex mediates monoubiquitination of FANCD2 but does not possess any Ub-conjugating activity. Very recently, the immunopurified FA complex was shown to contain PHD finger protein 9 (PHF9), which acts as an E3 ligase in vitro and is essential for FANCD2 monoubiquitination in vivo (Meetei et al. 2003) (Fig. 6b). The relevance of PHF9 to the FA complex is further under-

---

connected with "error-free" DNA-repair. **b** Monoubiquitin-mediated signaling in the Fanconi anemia (*FA*) pathway. BRCA2/D1 is the sensor on the DNA that, following damages, recruits the FA complex. This, in turn, monoubiquitinates FANCD2, through the action of one of its components, FANCL. This event allows the recruitment of monoubiquitinated FANCD2 to BRCA1- and RAD51-containing nuclear foci, which are sites of active DNA repair

scored by the fact that it identifies a previously uncharacterized complementation group in FA. PHF9 was in fact found defective in an individual
with a genetic defect that did not belong to any of the "canonical" complementation groups and was renamed, for this reason, FANCL (Meetei
et al. 2003).

Finally, the FA pathway is strictly interconnected with the BRCA
(breast cancer susceptibility gene) pathway. Indeed, BRCA2 was recently
identified as the FANCD1 gene (Howlett et al. 2002). Moreover, with siR-
NA silencing it was demonstrated that BRCA1 is required for targeting
FANCD2 to the site of DNA damage but is not responsible for FANCD2
monoubiquitination (Vandenberg et al. 2003). It has also been reported
that interaction between the two proteins occurs only with the ubiquitinated form of FANCD2 (Vandenberg et al. 2003). The molecular basis
for this targeting remains unclear, but it is likely to involve Ub receptors
at sites of DNA repair that await discovery.

8
Mono or Poly? An E3 Dilemma

8.1
Specificity Is Given by the E3 Ligase

A major unanswered question concerns how the Ub machinery makes
the decision whether to mono- or polyubiquitinate a substrate. One possibility is that different subsets of Ub ligases have specificity for the two
different modifications. For instance, p53 was shown to be regulated by
both mono- and polyubiquitination. Two different Ub ligases are involved: Mdm2 mediates monoubiquitination of p53 (Lai et al. 2001),
whereas p300-CBP promotes its polyubiquitination and proteasomal
degradation (Grossman et al. 2003). The Mms2-Ubc13 complex provides
an example of how specificity for polyubiquitination is achieved. This
UEV-E2 complex, as discussed above, is involved in postreplicative DNA
repair in yeast and was shown to assemble lysine 63-linked polyubiquitin chains in vitro. The crystal structure of the complex reveals that lysine 63 is exclusively used in chain assembly, most probably because the
relevant Ub binds in a way that other lysines are sterically excluded from
the E2 active site (VanDemark et al. 2001; McKenna, S. et al. 2003).

8.2
Specificity Is Given by the Substrate

In many cases, however, the same E3 enzyme is known to catalyze both mono- and polyubiquitination. An example of this is Cbl, which directs polyubiquitination and proteasomal degradation of cytoplasmic proteins, including Sprouty, Src, and Abl tyrosine kinases (Soubeyran et al. 2002; Yokouchi et al. 2001; Russell et al. 2000; Rubin et al. 2003), and monoubiquitination of RTKs and CIN85 (Haglund et al. 2003; Mosesson et al. 2003; Haglund et al. 2002). The same is true for Nedd4, which is able to act as a monoubiquitin-specific ligase on eps15 and Hrs (Polo et al. 2002; Katz et al. 2002) and is also able to polyubiquitinate intracellular substrates (Magnifico et al. 2003). Rsp5, the yeast homolog of Nedd4, can also mediate both modifications on different substrates (Dunn and Hicke 2001; Pickart 2001). How this dual specificity is achieved remains a mystery. One obvious possibility is that the same E3 ligase can enter different macromolecular complexes (also as a function of time and space in a given signaling pathway) that direct the catalytic specificity towards mono- or polyubiquitination.

Recent findings, however, suggest alternative, albeit not mutually exclusive, possibilities. Studies of UIMs and CUEs have revealed how these domains are endowed with a dual function of binding to Ub and being indispensable for monoubiquitination (Polo et al. 2002; Shih et al. 2002; Shih et al. 2003; Klapisz et al. 2002). Importantly, they do not contain lysines that function as acceptors of Ub, so their requirement for monoubiquitination must relate to different aspects of the process, most probably the recognition of Ub ligases (Polo et al. 2002). One possibility is that recognition between E3 and UIM- (or CUE)-containing proteins is mediated by the Ub that is present in the thiol-ester intermediate of E3. Once Ub is transferred to the substrate, the E3 ligase might dissociate, yielding a monoubiquitinated protein (Di Fiore et al. 2003; Polo et al. 2002). Alternatively, after ubiquitination, the intramolecular binding of UIMs (or CUEs) to Ub might sterically hinder the formation of Ub chains, as the major polyubiquitination site in Ub, lysine 48, is masked in both UIM-ubiquitin and CUE-ubiquitin complexes (Kang et al. 2003; Shekhtman Cowburn 2002). Such an "occlusion mechanism" might also be triggered by intermolecular Ub-Ub receptor interactions, thus providing a plausible explanation of why Cbl, known to direct polyubiquitination of other cellular proteins (Soubeyran et al. 2002; Rubin et al. 2003; Yokouchi et al. 1999), mediates solely monoubiquitination of RTKs and RTK-associated CIN85 (Haglund et al. 2003; Mosesson et al. 2003;

Haglund et al. 2003). In this case, binding of UIMs (or other domains) to monoubiquitinated RTKs might limit the elongation of Ub chains and thus cause predominant monoubiquitination of endocytic cargo proteins.

8.3
Balance Between E3 Ligases and Deubiquitinating Enzymes Determines Mono- Versus Polyubiquitination

Ubiquitination is a dynamic and reversible process, and the rapid removal of Ub is mediated by the activity of deubiquitinating enzymes (DUBs) (Wilkinson 2000). Deubiquitinating enzymes are constitutively active in the removal of Ub from substrates. It is therefore possible that a balance between activity and subcellular localization of DUBs and Ub ligases determines whether a specific protein becomes mono- or polyubiquitinated. Clearly, further experimental effort is needed to assess whether one or a combination of the outlined mechanisms determines the type of Ub modification in vivo and thus the fate and the function of Ub-tagged substrates.

9
Conclusions

Ubiquitin modification, in its various forms, constitutes a multifaceted regulation mechanism of fundamental importance to cellular homeostasis. As we start to appreciate the complexity of the system, many important questions come into focus. The first question is how ubiquitination, and in particular monoubiquitination, regulates protein function. The evidence reviewed here indicates that in many cases monoubiquitination should be regarded as a signaling post-translational modification that, much like phosphorylation, enables the signaling-dependent formation of dynamic networks of protein-protein interactions, thus allowing downstream propagation of the signal. Ubiquitination is, however, a bulky modification, and thus it is also projected to have impact *in cis* on protein function, for example, by regulating the activity of ubiquitinated enzymes. A second, and very important, question relates to the specificity of recognition between ubiquitinated proteins and Ub receptors. Although structural knowledge is being acquired on the modality of interaction between Ub and Ub-binding modules, the issue of specificity remains unsolved. Another facet of this problem relates to how Ub receptors discriminate between polyubiquitinated proteins, which are projected to be the vast majority of Ub-containing proteins in the cell, and monoubiquitinated proteins. Finally, because many E3 ligases are capable of both poly- and monoubiquitination, the issue of how the enzyme "decides" on the catalytic mode to operate is still rather obscure. Subversion of the Ub pathway plays a role in many diseases (D'Andrea 2003; Vu and Sakamoto 2000; Giasson and Lee 2003) ; given the profound impact of this modification on cellular physiology, it can be anticipated that the list is bound to grow. Our ability to harness and to modulate the system for therapeutic purposes will largely depend on providing answers to the above questions.

Acknowledgements The authors' work is supported by grants from Italian Association for Cancer Research (AIRC), Human Science Frontier Program, the International Association for Cancer Research (IARC), The European Community (VI Framework), the Telethon Foundation, and the Italian Ministry of Health.

References

Ahn, S. et al. Src-dependent tyrosine phosphorylation regulates dynamin self-assembly and ligand-induced endocytosis of the epidermal growth factor receptor. J Biol Chem 277, 26642–51 (2002)

Andoniou, C. E., Thien, C. B., Langdon, W. Y. Tumour induction by activated abl involves tyrosine phosphorylation of the product of the cbl oncogene. Embo J 13, 4515–23 (1994)

Andoniou, C. E. et al. The Cbl proto-oncogene product negatively regulates the Src-family tyrosine kinase Fyn by enhancing its degradation. Mol Cell Biol 20, 851–67 (2000)

Babst, M., Katzmann, D. J., Estepa-Sabal, E. J., Meerloo, T., Emr, S. D. Escrt-III: an endosome-associated heterooligomeric protein complex required for mvb sorting. Dev Cell 3, 271–82 (2002)

Babst, M., Katzmann, D. J., Snyder, W. B., Wendland, B., Emr, S. D. Endosome-associated complex, ESCRT-II, recruits transport machinery for protein sorting at the multivesicular body. Dev Cell 3, 283–9 (2002)

Bach, I., Ostendorff, H. P. Orchestrating nuclear functions: ubiquitin sets the rhythm. Trends Biochem Sci 28, 189–95 (2003)

Bache, K. G., Raiborg, C., Mehlum, A., Stenmark, H. STAM and Hrs are subunits of a multivalent Ubiquitin-binding complex on early endosomes. J Biol Chem (2003)

Baker, D., Hicke, L., Rexach, M., Schleyer, M., Schekman, R. Reconstitution of SEC gene product-dependent intercompartmental protein transport. Cell 54, 335–44 (1988)

Barbieri, M. A. et al. Epidermal growth factor and membrane trafficking. EGF receptor activation of endocytosis requires Rab5a. J Cell Biol 151, 539–50 (2000)

Bilodeau, P. S., Urbanowski, J. L., Winistorfer, S. C., Piper, R. C. The Vps27p Hse1p complex binds ubiquitin and mediates endosomal protein sorting. Nat Cell Biol 4, 534–9 (2002)

Bishop, N., Horman, A., Woodman, P. Mammalian class E vps proteins recognize ubiquitin and act in the removal of endosomal protein-ubiquitin conjugates. J Cell Biol 157, 91–101 (2002)

Brett, T. J., Traub, L. M., Fremont, D. H. Accessory protein recruitment motifs in clathrin-mediated endocytosis. Structure (Camb) 10, 797–809 (2002)

Briggs, S. D. et al. Gene silencing: trans-histone regulatory pathway in chromatin. Nature 418, 498 (2002)

Buchberger, A. From UBA to UBX: new words in the ubiquitin vocabulary. Trends Cell Biol 12, 216–21 (2002)

Burnett, B., Li, F., Pittman, R. N. The polyglutamine neurodegenerative protein ataxin-3 binds polyubiquitylated proteins and has ubiquitin protease activity. Hum Mol Genet (2003)

Carter, R. S., Geyer, B. C., Xie, M., Acevedo-Suarez, C. A., Ballard, D. W. Persistent activation of NF-kappa B by the tax transforming protein involves chronic phosphorylation of IkappaB kinase subunits IKKbeta and IKKgamma. J Biol Chem 276, 24445–8 (2001)

Carter, R. S., Pennington, K. N., Ungurait, B. J., Arrate, P., Ballard, D. W. Signal-induced ubiquitination of Ikappa B kinase-beta. J Biol Chem (2003)

Chen, H. et al. Epsin is an EH-domain-binding protein implicated in clathrin-mediated endocytosis. Nature 394, 793–7 (1998)

Courbard, J. R. et al. Interaction between two E3 ubiquitin ligases of different classes, CBLC and AIP4/ITCH. J Biol Chem 10, 10 (2002)

D'Andrea, A. D. The Fanconi road to cancer. Genes Dev 17, 1933–6 (2003)

D'Andrea, A. D., Grompe, M. The Fanconi anaemia/BRCA pathway. Nat Rev Cancer 3, 23–34 (2003)

Debonneville, C. et al. Phosphorylation of Nedd4–2 by Sgk1 regulates epithelial Na(+) channel cell surface expression. Embo J 20, 7052–9 (2001)

Delhase, M., Hayakawa, M., Chen, Y., Karin, M. Positive and negative regulation of IkappaB kinase activity through IKKbeta subunit phosphorylation. Science 284, 309–13 (1999)

de Melker, A. A., van der Horst, G., Calafat, J., Jansen, H., Borst, J. c-Cbl ubiquitinates the EGF receptor at the plasma membrane and remains receptor associated throughout the endocytic route. J Cell Sci 114, 2167–78. (2001)

de Winter, J. P. et al. The Fanconi anaemia group G gene FANCG is identical with XRCC9. Nat Genet 20, 281–3 (1998)

de Winter, J. P. et al. Isolation of a cDNA representing the Fanconi anemia complementation group E gene. Am J Hum Genet 67, 1306–8 (2000)

de Winter, J. P. et al. The Fanconi anemia protein FANCF forms a nuclear complex with FANCA, FANCC and FANCG. Hum Mol Genet 9, 2665–74 (2000)

Dieckmann, T. et al. Structure of a human DNA repair protein UBA domain that interacts with HIV-1 Vpr. Nat Struct Biol 5, 1042–7 (1998)

Di Fiore, P. P., Polo, S., Hofmann, K. When ubiquitin meets ubiquitin receptors: a signalling connection. Nat Rev Mol Cell Biol 4, 491–7 (2003)

Dikic, I. CIN85/CMS family of adaptor molecules. FEBS Lett 529, 110–5 (2002)

Dikic, I., Szymkiewicz, I., Soubeyran, P. Cbl signaling networks in the regulation of cell function. Cell Mol Life Sci 60, 1805–27 (2003)

Donaldson, K. M. et al. Ubiquitin-mediated sequestration of normal cellular proteins into polyglutamine aggregates. Proc Natl Acad Sci U S A 100, 8892–7 (2003)

Donaldson, K. M., Yin, H., Gekakis, N., Supek, F., Joazeiro, C. A. Ubiquitin Signals Protein Trafficking via Interaction with a Novel Ubiquitin Binding Domain in the Membrane Fusion Regulator, Vps9p. Curr Biol 13, 258–62 (2003)

Dover, J. et al. Methylation of histone H3 by COMPASS requires ubiquitination of histone H2B by Rad6. J Biol Chem 277, 28368–71 (2002)

Drake, M. T., Downs, M. A., Traub, L. M. Epsin binds to clathrin by associating directly with the clathrin-terminal domain. Evidence for cooperative binding through two discrete sites. J Biol Chem 275, 6479–89 (2000)

Duan, L. et al. Cbl-mediated ubiquitinylation is required for lysosomal sorting of epidermal growth factor receptor but is dispensable for endocytosis. J Biol Chem 278, 28950–60 (2003)

Dunn, R., Hicke, L. Multiple roles for Rsp5p-dependent ubiquitination at the internalization step of endocytosis. J Biol Chem 276, 25974–81 (2001)

Ekstrand, A. J., Sugawa, N., James, C. D., Collins, V. P. Amplified and rearranged epidermal growth factor receptor genes in human glioblastomas reveal deletions of sequences encoding portions of the N- and/or C-terminal tails. Proc Natl Acad Sci U S A 89, 4309–13 (1992)

Farsad, K. et al. Generation of high curvature membranes mediated by direct endophilin bilayer interactions. J Cell Biol 155, 193–200 (2001)

Fisher, R. D. et al. Structure and ubiquitin binding of the ubiquitin interacting motif. J Biol Chem 278, 28976–84 (2003)

Garcia-Higuera, I., Kuang, Y., D'Andrea, A. D. The molecular and cellular biology of Fanconi anemia. Curr Opin Hematol 6, 83–8 (1999)

Garrus, J. E. et al. Tsg101 and the vacuolar protein sorting pathway are essential for HIV-1 budding. Cell 107, 55–65 (2001)

Giasson, B. I., Lee, V. M. Are ubiquitination pathways central to Parkinson's disease? Cell 114, 1–8 (2003)

Grossman, S. R. et al. Polyubiquitination of p53 by a ubiquitin ligase activity of p300. Science 300, 342–4 (2003)

Gregory, R. C., Taniguchi, T., D'Andrea, A. D. Regulation of the Fanconi anemia pathway by monoubiquitination. Semin Cancer Biol 13, 77–82 (2003)

Haglund, K. et al. Multiple monoubiquitination of RTKs is sufficient for their endocytosis and degradation. Nat Cell Biol 5, 461–6 (2003)

Haglund, K., Shimokawa, N., Szymkiewicz, I., Dikic, I. Cbl-directed monoubiquitination of CIN85 is involved in regulation of ligand-induced degradation of EGF receptors. Proc Natl Acad Sci U S A 99, 12191–6 (2002)

Hama, H., Tall, G. G., Horazdovsky, B. F. Vps9p is a guanine nucleotide exchange factor involved in vesicle-mediated vacuolar protein transport. J Biol Chem 274, 15284–91 (1999)

Hershko, A., Ciechanover, A. The ubiquitin system. Annu Rev Biochem 67, 425–79 (1998)

Hicke, L. A new ticket for entry into budding vesicles-ubiquitin. Cell 106, 527–30 (2001)

Hicke, L. Protein regulation by monoubiquitin. Nat Rev Mol Cell Biol 2, 195–201 (2001)

Hinrichsen, L., Harborth, J., Andrees, L., Weber, K., Ungewickell, E. J. Effect of clathrin heavy chain- and alpha -adaptin specific small interfering RNAs on endocytic accessory proteins and receptor trafficking in HeLa cells. J Biol Chem (2003)

Hitchcock, A. L., Auld, K., Gygi, S. P., Silver, P. A. A subset of membrane-associated proteins is ubiquitinated in response to mutations in the endoplasmic reticulum degradation machinery. Proc Natl Acad Sci U S A 100, 12735–40 (2003)

Hoege, C., Pfander, B., Moldovan, G. L., Pyrowolakis, G., Jentsch, S. RAD6-dependent DNA repair is linked to modification of PCNA by ubiquitin and SUMO. Nature 419, 135–41 (2002)

Hofmann, K., Bucher, P. The UBA domain: a sequence motif present in multiple enzyme classes of the ubiquitination pathway. Trends Biochem Sci 21, 172–3 (1996)

Hofmann, K., Falquet, L. A ubiquitin-interacting motif conserved in components of the proteasomal and lysosomal protein degradation systems. Trends Biochem Sci 26, 347–50 (2001)

Hofmann, R. M., Pickart, C. M. Noncanonical MMS2-encoded ubiquitin-conjugating enzyme functions in assembly of novel polyubiquitin chains for DNA repair. Cell 96, 645–53 (1999)

Hook, S. S., Orian, A., Cowley, S. M., Eisenman, R. N. Histone deacetylase 6 binds polyubiquitin through its zinc finger (PAZ domain) and copurifies with deubiquitinating enzymes. Proc Natl Acad Sci U S A 99, 13425–30 (2002)

Horiuchi, H. et al. A novel Rab5 GDP/GTP exchange factor complexed to Rabaptin-5 links nucleotide exchange to effector recruitment and function. Cell 90, 1149–59 (1997)

Howlett, N. G. et al. Biallelic inactivation of BRCA2 in Fanconi anemia. Science 297, 606–9 (2002)

Hutchings, N. J., Clarkson, N., Chalkley, R., Barclay, A. N., Brown, M. H. Linking the T cell surface protein CD2 to the actin-capping protein CAPZ via CMS and CIN85. J Biol Chem 278, 22396–403 (2003)

Hwang, W. W. et al. A Conserved RING Finger Protein Required for Histone H2B Monoubiquitination and Cell Size Control. Mol Cell 11, 261–6 (2003)

Jiang, X., Huang, F., Marusyk, A., Sorkin, A. Grb2 Regulates Internalization of EGF Receptors through Clathrin-coated Pits. Mol Biol Cell 14, 858–70 (2003)

Jiang, X., Sorkin, A. Epidermal growth factor receptor internalization through clathrin-coated pits requires Cbl RING finger and proline-rich domains but not receptor polyubiquitylation. Traffic 4, 529–43 (2003)

Kang, R. S. et al. Solution structure of a CUE-ubiquitin complex reveals a conserved mode of ubiquitin binding. Cell 113, 621–30 (2003)

Katz, M. et al. Ligand-independent degradation of epidermal growth factor receptor involves receptor ubiquitylation and Hgs, an adaptor whose ubiquitin-interacting motif targets ubiquitylation by Nedd4. Traffic 3, 740–51 (2002)

Katzmann, D. J., Babst, M., Emr, S. D. Ubiquitin-dependent sorting into the multivesicular body pathway requires the function of a conserved endosomal protein sorting complex, ESCRT-I. Cell 106, 145–55 (2001)

Katzmann, D. J., Odorizzi, G., Emr, S. D. Receptor downregulation and multivesicular-body sorting. Nat Rev Mol Cell Biol 3, 893–905 (2002)

Kirsch, K. H. et al. The adapter type protein CMS/CD2AP binds to the proto-onco-genic protein c-Cbl through a tyrosine phosphorylation-regulated Src homology 3 domain interaction. J Biol Chem 276, 4957–63 (2001)

Klapisz, E. et al. A ubiquitin-interacting motif (UIM) is essential for Eps15 and Eps15R ubiquitination. J Biol Chem 277, 30746–53 (2002)

Komada, M., Soriano, P. Hrs, a FYVE finger protein localized to early endosomes, is implicated in vesicular traffic and required for ventral folding morphogenesis. Genes Dev 13, 1475–85 (1999)

Kowanetz, K. et al. Identification of a novel proline-arginine motif involved in CIN85-dependent clustering of Cbl and down-regulation of epidermal growth factor receptors. J Biol Chem 278, 39735–46 (2003)

Lafont, F., Simons, K. Raft-partitioning of the ubiquitin ligases Cbl and Nedd4 upon IgE- triggered cell signaling. Proc Natl Acad Sci U S A 98, 3180–4. (2001)

Lai, Z. et al. Human mdm2 mediates multiple mono-ubiquitination of p53 by a mechanism requiring enzyme isomerization. J Biol Chem 276, 31357–67 (2001)

Lee, P. S. et al. The Cbl protooncoprotein stimulates CSF-1 receptor multiubiquitina-tion and endocytosis, and attenuates macrophage proliferation. Embo J 18, 3616–28 (1999)

Levkowitz, G. et al. c-Cbl/Sli-1 regulates endocytic sorting and ubiquitination of the epidermal growth factor receptor. Genes Dev 12, 3663–74. (1998)

Levkowitz, G. et al. Ubiquitin ligase activity and tyrosine phosphorylation underlie suppression of growth factor signaling by c-Cbl/Sli-1. Mol Cell 4, 1029–40 (1999)

Li, L., Cohen, S. N. Tsg101: a novel tumor susceptibility gene isolated by controlled homozygous functional knockout of allelic loci in mammalian cells. Cell 85, 319–29 (1996)

Li, Q., Verma, I. M. NF-kappaB regulation in the immune system. Nat Rev Immunol 2, 725–34 (2002)

Lo Ten Foe, J. R. et al. Expression cloning of a cDNA for the major Fanconi anaemia gene, FAA. Nat Genet 14, 320–3 (1996)

Magnifico, A. et al. WW Domain HECT E3 s Target Cbl RING Finger E3 s for Protea-somal Degradation. J Biol Chem 278, 43169–77 (2003)

Mancini, A., Koch, A., Wilms, R., Tamura, T. c-Cbl associates directly with the C-ter-minal tail of the receptor for the macrophage colony-stimulating factor, c-Fms, and down-modulates this receptor but not the viral oncogene v-Fms. J Biol Chem 277, 14635–40. (2002)

McKenna, S. et al. Energetics and specificity of interactions within Ub.Uev.Ubc13 hu-man ubiquitin conjugation complexes. Biochemistry 42, 7922–30 (2003)

Meetei, A. R. et al. A novel ubiquitin ligase is deficient in Fanconi anemia. Nat Genet 35, 165–70 (2003)

Melchior, F. SUMO–nonclassical ubiquitin. Annu Rev Cell Dev Biol 16, 591–626 (2000)

Meyer, H. H., Wang, Y., Warren, G. Direct binding of ubiquitin conjugates by the mammalian p97 adaptor complexes, p47 and Ufd1-Npl4. Embo J 21, 5645–52 (2002)

Miyake, S., Lupher, M. L., Jr., Druker, B., Band, H. The tyrosine kinase regulator Cbl enhances the ubiquitination and degradation of the platelet-derived growth fac-tor receptor alpha. Proc Natl Acad Sci U S A 95, 7927–32 (1998)

Mochida, J., Yamamoto, T., Fujimura-Kamada, K., Tanaka, K. The novel adaptor protein, Mti1p, and Vrp1p, a homolog of Wiskott-Aldrich syndrome protein-interacting protein (WIP), may antagonistically regulate type I myosins in Saccharomyces cerevisiae. Genetics 160, 923–34 (2002)

Mosesson, Y. et al. Endocytosis of receptor tyrosine kinases is driven by monoubiquitylation, not polyubiquitylation. J Biol Chem 278, 21323–6 (2003)

Mori, S., Heldin, C. H., Claesson-Welsh, L. Ligand-induced ubiquitination of the platelet-derived growth factor beta-receptor plays a negative regulatory role in its mitogenic signaling. J Biol Chem 268, 577–83 (1993)

Motley, A., Bright, N. A., Seaman, M. N., Robinson, M. S. Clathrin-mediated endocytosis in AP-2-depleted cells. J Cell Biol 162, 909–18 (2003)

Mueller, T. D., Feigon, J. Solution structures of UBA domains reveal a conserved hydrophobic surface for protein-protein interactions. J Mol Biol 319, 1243–55 (2002)

Muller, S., Hoege, C., Pyrowolakis, G., Jentsch, S. SUMO, ubiquitin's mysterious cousin. Nat Rev Mol Cell Biol 2, 202–10 (2001)

Naar, A. M., Lemon, B. D., Tjian, R. Transcriptional coactivator complexes. Annu Rev Biochem 70, 475–501 (2001)

Nakatsu, F. et al. A Di-leucine signal in the ubiquitin moiety. Possible involvement in ubiquitination-mediated endocytosis. J Biol Chem 275, 26213–9 (2000)

Nyberg, K. A., Michelson, R. J., Putnam, C. W., Weinert, T. A. Toward maintaining the genome: DNA damage and replication checkpoints. Annu Rev Genet 36, 617–56 (2002)

Oldham, C. E., Mohney, R. P., Miller, S. L., Hanes, R. N., O'Bryan, J. P. The ubiquitin-interacting motifs target the endocytic adaptor protein epsin for ubiquitination. Curr Biol 12, 1112–6 (2002)

Ortolan, T. G. et al. The DNA repair protein rad23 is a negative regulator of multi-ubiquitin chain assembly. Nat Cell Biol 2, 601–8 (2000)

Peng, J. et al. A proteomics approach to understanding protein ubiquitination. Nat Biotechnol 21, 921–926 (2003)

Peschard, P. et al. Mutation of the c-Cbl TKB domain binding site on the Met receptor tyrosine kinase converts it into a transforming protein. Mol Cell 8, 995–1004. (2001)

Petrelli, A. et al. The endophilin-CIN85-Cbl complex mediates ligand-dependent downregulation of c-Met. Nature 416, 187–90. (2002)

Pham, A. D., Sauer, F. Ubiquitin-activating/conjugating activity of TAFII250, a mediator of activation of gene expression in Drosophila. Science 289, 2357–60 (2000)

Pickart, C. M. Ubiquitin in chains. Trends Biochem Sci 25, 544–8 (2000)

Pickart, C. M. Mechanisms underlying ubiquitination. Annu Rev Biochem 70, 503–33 (2001)

Piper, R. C., Cooper, A. A., Yang, H., Stevens, T. H. VPS27 controls vacuolar and endocytic traffic through a prevacuolar compartment in Saccharomyces cerevisiae. J Cell Biol 131, 603–17 (1995)

Polo, S. et al. A single motif responsible for ubiquitin recognition and monoubiquitination in endocytic proteins. Nature 416, 451–5 (2002)

Ponting, C. P. Proteins of the endoplasmic-reticulum-associated degradation pathway: domain detection and function prediction. Biochem J 351 Pt 2, 527–35 (2000)

Pornillos, O. et al. Structure and functional interactions of the Tsg101 UEV domain. Embo J 21, 2397–406 (2002)

Prag, G. et al. Mechanism of ubiquitin recognition by the CUE domain of Vps9p. Cell 113, 609–20 (2003)

Raiborg, C. et al. Hrs sorts ubiquitinated proteins into clathrin-coated microdomains of early endosomes. Nat Cell Biol 4, 394–8 (2002)

Rao, H., Sastry, A. Recognition of specific ubiquitin conjugates is important for the proteolytic functions of the ubiquitin-associated domain proteins Dsk2 and Rad23. J Biol Chem 277, 11691–5 (2002)

Ridge, S. A., Worwood, M., Oscier, D., Jacobs, A., Padua, R. A. FMS mutations in myelodysplastic, leukemic, and normal subjects. Proc Natl Acad Sci U S A 87, 1377–80 (1990)

Ringstad, N. et al. Endophilin/SH3p4 is required for the transition from early to late stages in clathrin-mediated synaptic vesicle endocytosis. Neuron 24, 143–54 (1999)

Robzyk, K., Recht, J., Osley, M. A. Rad6-dependent ubiquitination of histone H2B in yeast. Science 287, 501–4 (2000)

Rubin, C. et al. Sprouty fine-tunes EGF signaling through interlinked positive and negative feedback loops. Curr Biol 13, 297–307 (2003)

Russell, C. S., Ben-Yehuda, S., Dix, I., Kupiec, M., Beggs, J. D. Functional analyses of interacting factors involved in both pre-mRNA splicing and cell cycle progression in Saccharomyces cerevisiae. Rna 6, 1565–72 (2000)

Salcini, A. E., Chen, H., Iannolo, G., De Camilli, P., Di Fiore, P. P. Epidermal growth factor pathway substrate 15, Eps15. Int J Biochem Cell Biol 31, 805–9 (1999)

Sanjay, A., Horne, W. C., Baron, R. The Cbl family: ubiquitin ligases regulating signaling by tyrosine kinases. Sci STKE 2001, E40. (2001)

Schmidt, A. et al. Endophilin I mediates synaptic vesicle formation by transfer of arachidonate to lysophosphatidic acid. Nature 401, 133–41 (1999)

Schnell, J. D., Hicke, L. Non-traditional Functions of Ubiquitin and Ubiquitin-binding proteins. J Biol Chem (2003)

Seachrist, J. L. et al. Rab5 association with the angiotensin II type 1A receptor promotes Rab5 GTP binding and vesicular fusion. J Biol Chem 277, 679–85 (2002)

Seigneurin-Berny, D. et al. Identification of components of the murine histone deacetylase 6 complex: link between acetylation and ubiquitination signaling pathways. Mol Cell Biol 21, 8035–44 (2001)

Shekhtman, A., Cowburn, D. A ubiquitin-interacting motif from Hrs binds to and occludes the ubiquitin surface necessary for polyubiquitination in monoubiquitinated proteins. Biochem Biophys Res Commun 296, 1222–7 (2002)

Shih, S. C., Sloper-Mould, K. E., Hicke, L. Monoubiquitin carries a novel internalization signal that is appended to activated receptors. Embo J 19, 187–98 (2000)

Shih, S. C. et al. Epsins and Vps27p/Hrs contain ubiquitin-binding domains that function in receptor endocytosis. Nat Cell Biol 4, 389–93 (2002)

Shih, S. C. et al. A ubiquitin-binding motif required for intramolecular monoubiquitylation, the CUE domain. Embo J 22, 1273–81 (2003)

Shu, H. K., Pelley, R. J., Kung, H. J. Dissecting the activating mutations in v-erbB of avian erythroblastosis virus strain R. J Virol 65, 6173–80 (1991)

Snyder, P. M., Olson, D. R., Thomas, B. C. Serum and glucocorticoid-regulated kinase modulates Nedd4–2-mediated inhibition of the epithelial Na+ channel. J Biol Chem 277, 5–8 (2002)

Sorkin, A. Internalization of the epidermal growth factor receptor: role in signalling. Biochem Soc Trans 29, 480–4 (2001)

Soubeyran, P., Kowanetz, K., Szymkiewicz, I., Langdon, W. Y., Dikic, I. Cbl-CIN85-endophilin complex mediates ligand-induced downregulation of EGF receptors. Nature 416, 183–7. (2002)

Stang, E., Johannessen, L. E., Knardal, S. L., Madshus, I. H. Polyubiquitination of the epidermal growth factor receptor occurs at the plasma membrane upon ligand-induced activation. J Biol Chem 275, 13940–7 (2000)

Stelter, P., Ulrich, H. D. Control of spontaneous and damage-induced mutagenesis by SUMO and ubiquitin conjugation. Nature 425, 188–91 (2003)

Strathdee, C. A., Gavish, H., Shannon, W. R., Buchwald, M. Cloning of cDNAs for Fanconi's anaemia by functional complementation. Nature 358, 434 (1992)

Strous, G. J., Gent, J. Dimerization, ubiquitylation and endocytosis go together in growth hormone receptor function. FEBS Lett 529, 102–9 (2002)

Strous, G. J., van Kerkhof, P., Govers, R., Ciechanover, A., Schwartz, A. L. The ubiquitin conjugation system is required for ligand-induced endocytosis and degradation of the growth hormone receptor. Embo J 15, 3806–12. (1996)

Sun, S. C., Ballard, D. W. Persistent activation of NF-kappaB by the tax transforming protein of HTLV-1: hijacking cellular IkappaB kinases. Oncogene 18, 6948–58 (1999)

Sun, Z. W., Allis, C. D. Ubiquitination of histone H2B regulates H3 methylation and gene silencing in yeast. Nature 418, 104–8 (2002)

Swanson, K. A., Kang, R. S., Stamenova, S. D., Hicke, L., Radhakrishnan, I. Solution structure of Vps27 UIM-ubiquitin complex important for endosomal sorting and receptor downregulation. Embo J 22, 4597–606 (2003)

Szymkiewicz, I. et al. CIN85 Participates in Cbl-b-mediated Down-regulation of Receptor Tyrosine Kinases. J Biol Chem 277, 39666–72. (2002)

Taher, T. E. et al. c-Cbl Is Involved in Met Signaling in B Cells and Mediates Hepatocyte Growth Factor-Induced Receptor Ubiquitination. J Immunol 169, 3793–800. (2002)

Taniguchi, T., Dandrea, A. D. Molecular pathogenesis of fanconi anemia. Int J Hematol 75, 123–8 (2002)

Taniguchi, T. et al. S-phase-specific interaction of the Fanconi anemia protein, FANCD2, with BRCA1 and RAD51. Blood 100, 2414–20 (2002)

Taniguchi, T. et al. Convergence of the fanconi anemia and ataxia telangiectasia signaling pathways. Cell 109, 459–72 (2002)

Terrell, J., Shih, S., Dunn, R., Hicke, L. A function for monoubiquitination in the internalization of a G protein-coupled receptor. Mol Cell 1, 193–202 (1998)

Thien, C. B., Walker, F., Langdon, W. Y. RING finger mutations that abolish c-Cbl-directed polyubiquitination and downregulation of the EGF receptor are insufficient for cell transformation. Mol Cell 7, 355–65. (2001)

van Delft, S., Govers, R., Strous, G. J., Verkleij, A. J., van Bergen en Henegouwen, P. M. Epidermal growth factor induces ubiquitination of Eps15. J Biol Chem 272, 14013–6 (1997)

VanDemark, A. P., Hofmann, R. M., Tsui, C., Pickart, C. M., Wolberger, C. Molecular insights into polyubiquitin chain assembly: crystal structure of the Mms2/Ubc13 heterodimer. Cell 105, 711–20 (2001)

Vandenberg, C. J. et al. BRCA1-independent ubiquitination of FANCD2. Mol Cell 12, 247–54 (2003)

Volpicelli, L. A., Lah, J. J., Levey, A. I. Rab5-dependent trafficking of the m4 muscarinic acetylcholine receptor to the plasma membrane, early endosomes, and multivesicular bodies. J Biol Chem 276, 47590–8 (2001)

Vu, P. K., Sakamoto, K. M. Ubiquitin-mediated proteolysis and human disease. Mol Genet Metab 71, 261–6 (2000)

Wang, B. et al. Structure and ubiquitin interactions of the conserved zinc finger domain of Npl4. J Biol Chem 278, 20225–34 (2003)

Wang, Y., Yeung, Y. G., Stanley, E. R. CSF-1 stimulated multiubiquitination of the CSF-1 receptor and of Cbl follows their tyrosine phosphorylation and association with other signaling proteins. J Cell Biochem 72, 119–34 (1999)

Wang, Y. et al. Negative regulation of EphA2 receptor by Cbl. Biochem Biophys Res Commun 296, 214–20. (2002)

Watanabe, S. et al. Characterization of the CIN85 adaptor protein and identification of components involved in CIN85 complexes. Biochem Biophys Res Commun 278, 167–74 (2000)

Waterman, H. et al. A mutant EGF-receptor defective in ubiquitylation and endocytosis unveils a role for Grb2 in negative signaling. Embo J 21, 303–13 (2002)

Wilde, A. et al. EGF receptor signaling stimulates SRC kinase phosphorylation of clathrin, influencing clathrin redistribution and EGF uptake. Cell 96, 677–87 (1999)

Wilkinson, C. R. et al. Proteins containing the UBA domain are able to bind to multi-ubiquitin chains. Nat Cell Biol 3, 939–43 (2001)

Wilkinson, K. D. Ubiquitination and deubiquitination: targeting of proteins for degradation by the proteasome. Semin Cell Dev Biol 11, 141–8. (2000)

Wong, A. et al. FRS2 alpha attenuates FGF receptor signaling by Grb2-mediated recruitment of the ubiquitin ligase Cbl. Proc Natl Acad Sci U S A 99, 6684–9. (2002)

Wood, A. et al. Bre1, an E3 ubiquitin ligase required for recruitment and substrate selection of Rad6 at a promoter. Mol Cell 11, 267–74 (2003)

Yokouchi, M. et al. Ligand-induced ubiquitination of the epidermal growth factor receptor involves the interaction of the c-Cbl RING finger and UbcH7. J Biol Chem 274, 31707–12. (1999)

Yokouchi, M. et al. Src-catalyzed phosphorylation of c-Cbl leads to the interdependent ubiquitination of both proteins. J Biol Chem 276, 35185–93. (2001)

Zandi, E., Karin, M. Bridging the gap: composition, regulation, and physiological function of the IkappaB kinase complex. Mol Cell Biol 19, 4547–51 (1999)

Subject Index

Current Topics in Microbiology and Immunology

Volumes published since 1989 (and still available)

Vol. 264/I: **Hacker, Jörg; Kaper, James B. (Eds.):** Pathogenicity Islands and the Evolution of Microbes. 2002. 34 figs. XVIII, 232 pp. ISBN 3-540-42681-7

Vol. 264/II: **Hacker, Jörg; Kaper, James B. (Eds.):** Pathogenicity Islands and the Evolution of Microbes. 2002. 24 figs. XVIII, 228 pp. ISBN 3-540-42682-5

Vol. 265: **Dietzschold, Bernhard; Richt, Jürgen A. (Eds.):** Protective and Pathological Immune Responses in the CNS. 2002. 21 figs. X, 278 pp. ISBN 3-540-42668-X

Vol. 266: **Cooper, Koproski (Eds.):** The Interface Between Innate and Acquired Immunity, 2002, 15 figs. XIV, 116 pp. ISBN 3-540-42894-1

Vol. 267: **Mackenzie, John S.; Barrett, Alan D. T.; Deubel, Vincent (Eds.):** Japanese Encephalitis and West Nile Viruses. 2002. 66 figs. X, 418 pp. ISBN 3-540-42783-X

Vol. 268: **Zwickl, Peter; Baumeister, Wolfgang (Eds.):** The Proteasome-Ubiquitin Protein Degradation Pathway. 2002, 17 figs. X, 213 pp. ISBN 3-540-43096-2

Vol. 269: **Koszinowski, Ulrich H.; Hengel, Hartmut (Eds.):** Viral Proteins Counteracting Host Defenses. 2002, 47 figs. XII, 325 pp. ISBN 3-540-43261-2

Vol. 270: **Beutler, Bruce; Wagner, Hermann (Eds.):** Toll-Like Receptor Family Members and Their Ligands. 2002, 31 figs. X, 192 pp. ISBN 3-540-43560-3

Vol. 271: **Koehler, Theresa M. (Ed.):** Anthrax. 2002, 14 figs. X, 169 pp. ISBN 3-540-43497-6

Vol. 272: **Doerfler, Walter; Böhm, Petra (Eds.):** Adenoviruses: Model and Vectors in Virus-Host Interactions. Virion and Structure, Viral Replication, Host Cell Interactions. 2003, 63 figs., approx. 280 pp. ISBN 3-540-00154-9

Vol. 273: **Doerfler, Walter; Böhm, Petra (Eds.):** Adenoviruses: Model and Vectors in Virus-Host Interactions. Immune System, Oncogenesis, Gene Therapy. 2004, 35 figs., approx. 280 pp. ISBN 3-540-06851-1

Vol. 274: **Workman, Jerry L. (Ed.):** Protein Complexes that Modify Chromatin. 2003, 38 figs., XII, 296 pp. ISBN 3-540-44208-1

Vol. 275: **Fan, Hung (Ed.):** Jaagsiekte Sheep Retrovirus and Lung Cancer. 2003, 63 figs., XII, 252 pp. ISBN 3-540-44096-3

Vol. 276: **Steinkasserer, Alexander (Ed.):** Dendritic Cells and Virus Infection. 2003, 24 figs., X, 296 pp. ISBN 3-540-44290-1

Vol. 277: **Rethwilm, Axel (Ed.):** Foamy Viruses. 2003, 40 figs., X, 214 pp. ISBN 3-540-44388-6

Vol. 278: **Salomon, Daniel R.; Wilson, Carolyn (Eds.):** Xenotransplantation. 2003, 22 figs., IX, 254 pp.ISBN 3-540-00210-3

Vol. 279: **Thomas, George; Sabatini, David; Hall, Michael N. (Eds.):** TOR. 2004, 49 figs., X, 364 pp.ISBN 3-540-00534-X

Vol. 280: **Heber-Katz, Ellen (Ed.):** Regeneration: Stem Cells and Beyond. 2004, 42 figs., XII, 194 pp.ISBN 3-540-02238-4

Vol. 281: **Young, John A. T. (Ed.):** Cellular Factors Involved in Early Steps of Retroviral Replication. 2003, 21 figs., IX, 240 pp. ISBN 3-540-00844-6

Vol. 282: **Stenmark, Harald (Ed.):** Phosphoinositides in Subcellular Targeting and Enzyme Activation. 2003, 20 figs., X, 210 pp. ISBN 3-540-00950-7

Vol. 283: **Kawaoka, Yoshihiro (Ed.):** Biology of Negative Strand RNA Viruses: The Power of Reverse Genetics. 2004, 24 figs., IX, 350 pp. ISBN 3-540-40661-1

Vol. 284: **Harris, David (Ed.):** Mad Cow Disease and Related Spongiform Encephalopathies. 2004, 34 figs., IX, 219 pp. ISBN 3-540-20107-6

Vol. 285: **Marsh, Mark (Ed.):** Membrane Trafficking in Viral Replication. 2004, 19 figs., approx, 270 pp. ISBN 3-540-21430-5